Surviving and Thriving: Your 1st Job as an RN

By Brenda Brozek, MAOL, RN
and Patricia McFarland, MS, RN, FAAN

Cover design by Jessica Bloom
Content design by Dena Fisher

Forewords by Mary Foley, PhD, RN, FAAN
and Ginger Manss, MSN, RN, AOCN

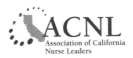

ACNL
Association of California
Nurse Leaders

Produced by Association of California Nurse Leaders
Endorsed by California Nursing Students' Association

Surviving and Thriving: Your 1st Job as an RN

Published by:
Association of California Nurse Leaders
2520 Venture Oaks Way, Suite 210
Sacramento, CA 95833

To order additional books, buy in bulk, order for corporate use, request a review copy for course adoption, request author information or for speaker or other media requests, contact the Association of California Nurse Leaders at 916.779.6949, or info@acnl.org.

ISBN: 978-1-4675-8779-2

Printed in the United States of America by Paul Baker Printing

To the students who inspire us, our colleagues who believe in us and our families for their support, love and encouragement!

And to newly licensed RNs...the future of our profession!

Acknowledgements

We are very grateful to the many people who helped make this book a reality:

Ginger Manss, from the beginning of this project your support never wavered. Thank you for your enthusiasm and belief in us and your commitment to the next generation of nurse leaders.

Members of the ACNL Board of Directors, thank you for committing the resources to bring this project to fruition.

Katie Lenihan, our chief volunteer, you helped with so many aspects of this book – especially as our deadline was fast approaching.

Kathy Harren and Mary Foley, you are inspirations to both of us. Thank you for being thought leaders whose shoulders we stand on.

Dena Fisher, your perseverance and skills in designing and laying-out the book's contents, even through all the edits, were invaluable to us.

Jessica Bloom, you created a beautiful design for our book cover.

Elizabeth Brozek, thank you for creating the book's charts and graphics – mostly on short notice.

Beth Gardner, for your vision and passion in supporting the next generation of RNs.

Wendy Smolich and Brian Carrick for all the behind the scenes work you do for us.

Thank you to those who provided insights and input for *Surviving and Thriving*:

Andrew Brozek
Suzette Cardin
Candy Collins
Kay Evans
Julie Feld
Kimberly Horton

Gwen Matthews
Stephanie Mearns
Robyn Nelson
Susan Odegaard Turner
Allen Orsi

And thank you to all the RNs who shared their stories for *Surviving and Thriving*. Read their stories beginning on page 171.

Patricia would also like to acknowledge:

My husband, Rick, whose love, encouragement and support has allowed me to pursue my dreams...

My parents who instilled in us that education opens doors. It was my honor and privilege to use all my nursing skills to make their last days more comfortable.

Katie, my sister and friend – my consummate cheerleader!

My co-author, Brenda Brozek, you invited me to join you in this new journey – what a ride we have had. You are a gifted communicator, collaborator and writer. Thank you!

To my mentors Ellen Frank, Maria O'Rourke, Margaret Mette and Deloras Jones. I carry you all in my heart – thank you!

Brenda would also like to acknowledge:

My husband, John, you inspire me each day! Thank you for your love and support.

My children, Andy and Lizzie – I'm very proud of both of you!

My co-author, Pat McFarland, you always look for the potential in others – thank you for seeing mine! It was a pleasure collaborating with you to write this book.

My cousin, Susan, you're my sister and role model.

My dear friend, Catherine, you're always there when I need you.

And the *Zine Women*, my mother and aunts – you believed in me and taught me that anything is possible. I think about you every day!

Table of Contents

Foreword   9
The Wonder of Nursing, by Mary Foley
Beginning Your Journey as an RN, by Ginger Manss

Introduction   13
Your Adventure in Nursing: Thriving in Your RN Career

Chapter 1   17
What to Expect: Your Growth as a Professional Nurse

Chapter 2   29
Paving the Road: Preceptors, Mentors and Role Models

Chapter 3   41
Defining Your Role as an RN: Important Resources
to Guide Your Practice

Chapter 4   63
Communication Skills: The Foundation of Your Success as an RN

Chapter 5   87
Effective Communication: Strategies for Challenging Situations

Chapter 6   115
Delegation: Empowerment and Accountability

Chapter 7   123
Opportunity or Uncertainty: Successfully Managing Change

Chapter 8   135
Quality and Patient Safety: You Can Make a Difference!

Chapter 9   157
Endless Possibilities: Looking Beyond Your 1st Job

Celebrating Nursing   171
Stories from RNs who travelled before you

Introduction   173
The Essence of Nursing, by Margarita Baggett

The Art of Nursing   177

Our Patients: Forever in Our Hearts   199

Our Preceptors and Mentors   225

The Health Care Team: Together We're Stronger   243

Finding Your Path   255

Afterword   277
Putting It All Together: Thriving as an RN

Glossary of Terms   283

Acronyms   286

References and Resources   287

My Notes...   295

Foreword

The Wonder of Nursing

Welcome to the profession of nursing and your first job as an RN! Thank you for the hard work you have already accomplished to reach this point in your life.

You are about to begin a career that will bring you the wonder of birth, the trauma of illness, the sadness of death and all the stages experienced in between. As nurses, we are privileged to be with people at these special times in their lives. Through our educational preparation, competency and compassion, we make a positive impact on patients, families and communities. Each year, nurses are held in the highest regard in the US as measured by the *Gallup Poll* – and nearly three million RNs work each day to make sure we earn that trust.

As you start your first job, you probably have many questions and concerns, and maybe even some self-doubt. This is one of the most special realities about nurses – throughout our careers, we will always have much to learn.

Your journey on the path of lifelong learning is about to begin. This book is intended for you at this special time in your career. The authors have provided you with the knowledge, tools and resources you need to help you survive and thrive. Be sure to read and reflect on the stories submitted by RN colleagues who have walked in your footsteps. As professionals, many of our greatest learnings come from sharing our stories and experiences.

Thank you again for joining the proud profession of nursing. I hope we meet someday in one of the great professional organizations that represent the many facets of our profession. As you enter this wonderful new world, I want to share a brief message with you from one of our most contemporary nurse leaders (after Ms. Nightingale, of course).

Dr. Margretta Styles was an educator and leader in nursing and was president of both the American Nurses Association and the International Council of Nurses. She left us many gifts, and one of her last messages about the importance of nurses guides my work each and every day.

"Imagine a world without nurses. Think of a world without persons who know what nurses know; who believe as nurses believe; who do what nurses do; who have the effect that nurses have on the health of individuals, families and the nation; who enjoy the trust that nurses enjoy from the American people. Imagine a world like that, a world without nurses."

I can't imagine such a world! Thank you Brenda and Pat for writing *Surviving and Thriving: Your 1st Job as an RN* to help launch the careers of nurses for generations to come.

Mary Foley, PhD, RN, FAAN
Director, Center for Nursing Research and Innovation
University of California, San Francisco
Past President, American Nurses Association

Foreword

Beginning Your Journey as an RN

Your first year as a Registered Nurse! All at once it can be exciting, terrifying, crazy, heartbreaking, confusing, satisfying, wonderful, exhausting and fulfilling.

There are times when you will make a mistake and worry that you have caused someone harm. There are other times when you will try your best, but wonder to yourself, "What did I do all day?" And there will be moments when you get that smile from a special patient – they grab your hand and hold it, or they tell you that you were the BEST nurse they ever had.

Those are the times when you know that you were born to be a nurse!

As you read this book, take time to think about the value of nursing – what a difference nurses make for our patients, clients, families and communities. Think about the nurses you know who give their all to deliver wonderful care.

If you are a new graduate reading this book, take it a chapter at a time. Know that each experience you have with patients will teach you something about yourself and your world. Give yourself time to learn. Utilize your resources, colleagues and friends to help you improve your practice and move to the next level of nursing.

If you are a nurse who is contemplating leaving our profession, read this book carefully to rediscover why you became a nurse in the first place. Maybe you're not in the right organization, the appropriate specialty or the best place for you to thrive. Use this book to help plan a new strategy to find your passion in nursing.

If you are not a nurse, but think that nursing may be your calling, we hope this book will help you understand the role of the professional nurse. You may wonder: Do people really talk about those things at lunch? Why would anyone love to do that? What is nursing all about anyway? *Surviving and Thriving: Your 1st Job as an RN* provides insight into this wonderful and rewarding profession, especially through the poignant stories from nurses that are included in this book.

Nursing is all encompassing. We touch people's lives when they are most vulnerable. We are present to celebrate the miracle of birth and ease the transition to death; to heal and to help people maximize their health. Nursing has touched my family for generations. I'm very proud to have followed my mother's footsteps into nursing and that my daughter Jennifer has followed mine.

The Association of California Nurse Leaders published *Surviving and Thriving: Your 1st Job as an RN* because we believe in investing in the future of our profession. ACNL seeks to develop and educate nurses along the continuum through our vision of creating and influencing the future of health care. *Surviving and Thriving* is a tool to help nurses maximize their potential – not only in the clinical aspects of patient care, but also in their development as effective team members, communicators and advocates.

As nurse leaders we hope this book inspires and ignites your passion for nursing as you begin your journey in this wonderful profession!

Ginger Manss, MSN, RN, AOCN
Director, Cancer Services/Telemetry/ICU
St. Joseph's Medical Center
Stockton, California
2012 President, Association of California Nurse Leaders

Introduction

Your Adventure in Nursing: Thriving in Your RN Career

Beginning your journey as a registered nurse is indeed exciting! You worked so hard to get here. You completed a challenging curriculum in nursing school and passed the licensing exam. You secured an RN position in a highly competitive job market. Now, you're ready to begin your career. Welcome to nursing!

Nursing is a rewarding and energizing profession. In this beginning phase of your career, you'll enter a new level of challenges, experiences and opportunities. Many of you will feel exhilarated and eager, but at the same time nervous and apprehensive. This is completely normal.

Although nursing school provided patient care experiences and exposure to hospitals and other health care work settings, many new graduate RNs feel overwhelmed and unprepared to cope with the challenges of their new careers as nurses. Some don't have clear or realistic expectations of their roles as registered nurses. As a result, of the nurses who leave our profession, many do so in their first year of practice.

Surviving and Thriving was created to be a resource for new graduates, nursing students and experienced RNs, as well as those interested in learning more about the nursing profession. This book will help you develop clear expectations about your role as a nurse and provides you with the knowledge and resources to successfully meet the challenges you'll face as a new RN.

Surviving and Thriving will help you:

    • Set realistic expectations of your learning and development as you move from novice to expert in nursing.

• Develop a clear understanding of your legal and ethical responsibilities as a professional nurse.

• Build strong communication skills – the foundation of your success as a caregiver, patient advocate and productive team member.

• Help ensure your success through optimal relationships with preceptors and mentors.

• Influence quality care and patient safety in your nursing practice.

• Prepare for the challenges of the rapidly changing health care environment.

• Take care of yourself to prevent compassion fatigue.

• Plot your career path beyond your first job.

The information in *Surviving and Thriving* is based on: extensive review of books and literature on key topics for new nurses; interviews and discussions with RNs at varying levels of experience who shared their knowledge and wisdom with us; and our experiences – which collectively represent more than 60 years in the nursing profession.

Although we've followed very different career paths, both your authors share a love of nursing and a strong desire to help the next generation of nurses find success in our profession.

Pat became an RN at the age of 20, and has been a nurse for nearly 40 years. She is a geriatric clinical nurse specialist by education, and has held varying positions in both acute and post-acute care. Pat has been a nursing administrator for many years and is currently CEO of a statewide professional nursing organization.

Brenda is a second career RN with a background in journalism and marketing. After working in cardiac care for several years, she became a nurse educator and later manager in a large staff development department. She is now a communication and education consultant, blending both her communication and nursing backgrounds.

In this book we're very proud to feature more than 40 stories from nurses who relate their experiences from their early careers as RNs. These inspiring narratives reveal the essence of nursing and the common bonds we nurses share.

We've also included a glossary to familiarize you with key terms and acronyms you'll hear in your RN role. At the end of each chapter, you'll find questions for reflection to help you solidify key concepts and apply them to your nursing practice.

Surviving and Thriving is meant to be a resource for you. A guide that not only provides information and tips, but is also a vehicle for reflection as you begin your career as an RN. As a new nurse, you may be wondering how you will improve your skills and competence, effectively care for your patients, become a productive team member and design a career that's right for you. It's our desire that this book will help you answer these and many other questions.

Although we've followed different paths in nursing, we have attained tremendous happiness, joy and fulfillment from our chosen careers. Nursing is a profession like no other. We wish you much success as you embark on your own personal journey as a registered nurse!

Patricia McFarland, MS, RN, FAAN
Brenda Brozek, MAOL, RN

What to Expect:
Your Growth as a Professional Nurse

*"Neither competence nor compassion is learned from a book.
They are behaviors – characteristic of professional practice."*

Leah Curtin, MS, MA, RN, FAAN

As you begin your career by securing your first job as a registered nurse, you're probably experiencing a mixture of excitement, anticipation and apprehension. You may be afraid that you aren't knowledgeable or experienced enough for your new role as an RN. This feeling can be especially strong when you observe or compare yourself to other nurses on your unit who seem to possess so much knowledge and expertise.

Rest assured, this is a common concern among new RNs. In her article, *From Student to Practicing Nurse*, Mary Ellis Smith summed up this feeling by saying: "Many new nurses feel that they've gone from being the smartest person in their class to being incompetent."

But think about how far you've come! You've completed the grueling nursing school curriculum and either passed the National Council Licensure Examination (NCLEX) or are preparing to take the exam. You've come a long way since that first day of nursing school. Yes, you still have a lot to learn! Your employer and fellow team members recognize that your journey is just beginning. Give yourself time to learn and grow.

"As a nurse you are often holding another person's life in your hands, but as a new grad you aren't always sure what to do with it." Jennifer Perisho

Read Jennifer's story, *10 Tips for New Grads*, on page 179.

Depending on the strategy your employer utilizes to educate and orient new graduate RNs, you'll have additional training and education, one or more nurse preceptors to guide you in the patient care area, as well as resources and support to help you successfully integrate into your new role.

No one expects you to have all the answers. As in many other professions, mastery of your role as a nurse occurs over time as you experience an increasing variety of patient care situations and build your knowledge, skills and confidence.

In her groundbreaking book, *From Novice to Expert,* Patricia Benner identified five stages that registered nurses move through as they transition from new nurse to expert nurse. You may have studied these stages in nursing school, but they take on new meaning as you begin your nursing career.

Benner also provides a generalized timeline for moving through these stages of development. However, this should be considered a guideline that varies depending on the individual. Also remember that this is a continuum – you don't magically pop from one phase to another. *Poof!* Yesterday I was a novice and when I woke up this morning I could feel that I'm now an advanced beginner. It doesn't work that way. Instead, the progression occurs over time as you gradually begin practicing at increasingly advanced levels.

Stages of Development

Stage 1: Novice *(1st Year of Practice)*

Beginners have little first-hand or experiential knowledge of the situations they're about to face. To give them a context for nursing practice, they initially learn about and focus on objective information, such as temperature, blood pressure, heart rate, oxygen saturation level, intake and output, etc. They learn rules about these measurements: diastolic blood pressure should be between 60 and 80, urine output should average at least 30 cc per hour, heart rate should be 60-100, and the list of rules goes on.

These rules guide action as the novice observes the disease processes impacting these rules and, as a result, the patient's condition. Benner cautions, however, that strictly following rules usually doesn't help the novice determine the most relevant tasks in a given situation. Gaining this contextual knowledge occurs as the beginner actually experiences a variety of clinical situations and has other nurses to guide them and help them interpret what they're seeing and experiencing.

Also in this phase, the novice is very focused on tasks and basic skills. Mastering skills such as starting IVs, drawing blood and inserting Foley catheters are concrete tasks that help the beginner build confidence as their ability to perform these skills increases.

Stage 2: Advanced Beginner *(1-2 years of practice)*

Advanced beginners have experienced enough clinical situations to understand and put meaning to the data and information they're observing and assimilating. Benner asserts that although nurses at this level still need support and continue to be concrete and task-focused, they can now recognize aspects and characteristics in their patients that can only be identified through prior experience and observation. They begin to link cause and effect, for example, correlating a patient's pale, cold, clammy skin with their sudden drop in heart rate and blood pressure.

Stage 3: Competent *(2-3 years of practice)*

According to Benner, "conscious, deliberate planning" is characteristic of this level of skill as the RN evolves from reacting to situations and performing tasks to synchronizing their knowledge and skills into a long-range plan of care for each patient. They can transfer the knowledge gained from one patient's situation to other patients. At this stage, it's also easier to prioritize work and determine what interventions are most important depending on the patient's needs and condition. Generally speaking, the competent nurse will still be striving to build speed and efficiency, but at the same time feels much more comfortable with their ability to cope with situations and the unforeseeable challenges that may arise during their shift.

Stage 4: Proficient *(3-5 years of practice)*

At the proficient level, the nurse has the ability to perceive situations as a whole and relate them to long-term goals. Benner explains that the proficient nurse knows from experience what typical events to expect in a given situation and how to modify plans and actions to respond to those events in order to keep the patient on track.

Nurses at this stage have evolved to a level where they can recognize when a patient isn't following a normal progression for their condition. As a result, the plan of care is adjusted to keep the patient moving forward toward their goals, whether it be discharge, independent self care, pain control, etc. The nurse at the proficient level now recognizes and interprets nuances in each situation that would be difficult for RNs in previous stages of development to interpret and apply.

"Each day in nursing, you can only give your very best to the patient in front of you – whatever your best may be at this stage in your career!" Ginger Manss

Read Ginger's story, *Give Yourself Time to Learn,* on page 196.

Stage 5: Expert *(More than 5 years of practice)*

This is the highest level of the continuum. Expert nurses have been exposed to so many patient care situations and experiences that they rarely problem-solve by using the analytical rules and tools they learned in the beginning stages. Instead, through their vast background of experience, they intuitively know how to respond in situations they are familiar with.

When working with an expert nurse, you may hear a conversation with the physician such as this: "I've taken care of Mr. Jones for three days, and I know there's something wrong. Even though his vitals are normal, he's just not the same."

An astute physician will often listen to the concerns of the intuitive expert nurse. We've seen many examples in our careers of physicians heeding these warnings and after examining the patient and/or ordering diagnostic tests, discovering there was indeed a problem or condition that, if left unchecked, could result in a negative outcome for the patient.

The Stages of Novice to Expert Aren't Just for New Nurses

It's important to note that Benner's stages of development aren't a once-in-a-career occurrence. Even experienced RNs will find themselves as novices or advanced beginners when significantly changing roles in nursing, and must learn a new skill set and context base for this new role. For example, RNs who transfer from med/surg to critical care or from staff positions to management roles, will find themselves back at the novice stage as they acclimate to their new positions.

To guide you through this process, it's important to have an excellent preceptor. As you move through your career, preceptors and mentors will be invaluable in providing wisdom and guidance and will challenge you to achieve your best. We'll discuss your relationship with preceptors and mentors in our next chapter.

Moving through the Stages of Novice to Expert

Brenda shares this story:

One night, in my role as relief charge nurse on a high acuity telemetry unit, I entered a patient's room to check on Karen, one of our newer RNs who had recently completed her new grad orientation. Her patient had a history of congestive heart failure and appeared to be mildly short of breath. I auscultated his chest and heard rales in his lower lobes. The patient was already on oxygen, and his O_2 saturation was lower than the last measurement recorded two hours prior.

I had Karen listen to his lungs and then took her into the hallway. I said that we needed to act immediately or he'd soon be in acute respiratory distress with pulmonary edema. I suggested that she call the physician to get a diuretic ordered and ask respiratory therapy to evaluate the patient. Karen looked at me questioningly and said: "Do you really think it's that bad? He seems comfortable to me. I think we should wait and see if it gets worse before we call the doctor."

I explained to her that we couldn't wait – we needed to be proactive. Karen called the MD and obtained orders for a diuretic and other interventions. In the short time it took Karen to obtain and administer IV Lasix, the fluid in the patient's lungs had increased, and he was no longer comfortable. Fortunately, his condition reversed quickly after the diuretic and a respiratory treatment.

Karen apologized to me for not knowing the patient was headed for trouble. But I explained that she had never seen a patient in the early stages of pulmonary edema. I didn't recognize the symptoms in my first patient, either. A more experienced RN helped me through it, just like I was helping her. Since then, I've seen many such patients. As a result, I can usually spot the symptoms early.

A few weeks later, Karen had another patient with similar symptoms. Because she had already experienced a patient in respiratory distress, she quickly recognized the problem. This time Karen acted quickly and another patient avoided an emergent situation.

Building Your Skills, Knowledge and Competency

As you begin your journey as a novice nurse, there are many strategies you can utilize to build your knowledge and skills, and as a result, your confidence. We discuss some of these strategies in this section. You'll learn other tips from your preceptor and nursing colleagues.

"...if a genuine commitment of care, respect, compassion and presence is made to the patient, you can and will be a wonderful nurse on day one!" Laura Giambattista

Read Laura's story, *It's Much More than Technical Skills*, on page 219.

Ask Questions

The simplest way to expand your knowledge base is to ask questions. Your colleagues on the health care team represent a wealth of information, expertise and know-how. Use these resources to help you expand your knowledge. Although you'll predominately be learning from your preceptor and other RNs in your department, don't limit your inquiries only to your fellow RNs. You can also learn a lot from physicians, respiratory care practitioners, pharmacists, physical therapists and other members of the health care team.

You may be thinking: *those people are too busy to talk to me, especially the physicians!* In reality, many MDs like to teach and are open to answering your questions about their patients' diagnoses and medical procedures. The same is true of other clinicians such as respiratory care practitioners, pharmacists, etc. Many are happy to share their knowledge and are flattered and appreciative that you're interested in their expertise. This will also help you build positive relationships with these health care team members. Once you start asking questions, you'll quickly identify those who enjoy sharing their knowledge. These are the professionals you can go back to when you have more questions.

Sometimes new RNs are afraid that if they ask too many questions, their colleagues might think they're incompetent. Just the opposite is true. Many RNs have told us they expect questions from new nurses. Conversely, those who ***don't*** ask questions are much more of a concern to them.

Asking Questions to Expand Your Knowledge

Brenda shares this story:

Felicia, a new hire RN with two years experience, was working on our night shift. As her preceptor for unit orientation, I found that she asked me very few questions about patient care on our unit. As she began working on her own, other RNs commented that Felicia rarely asked for advice or guidance and they were concerned.

One night, we noticed that Felicia was spending a significant amount of time with a post-op patient with a transurethral resection of the prostate (TURP). This wasn't a typical patient we cared for on our cardiac unit, but due to his history of coronary artery disease, he was sent to us. Because I was charge nurse, I asked Felicia several times if there was a problem, and each time she said no. However, I noticed that she called the MD twice and was giving the patient the maximum doses of his prn IV Morphine.

I assessed the patient and found that he was in severe pain and his lower abdomen was extremely distended. I noticed his Foley catheter bag was empty. Because I hadn't cared for many TURP patients, I asked a more experienced RN to assess him, over Felicia's objections. The other nurse confirmed what I suspected – due to bleeding and trauma from surgery, the patient's urinary catheter had become clogged with blood clots. When we irrigated the patient's catheter, the Foley bag filled with about 1000 mls of urine and he experienced nearly instant pain relief.

If Felicia had conferred with another RN on her team, her patient's pain would have been alleviated much sooner, he wouldn't have needed Morphine and the physician wouldn't have been called two times. Much more far-reaching, her team members were now very concerned about Felicia's unwillingness to collaborate with her colleagues about patient care issues.

The bottom line: If you don't know, ASK! This will help you increase your knowledge and skills, and most importantly, will help you provide the best care possible for your patients.

Read and Study

You can greatly expand your knowledge base and connect your patient care experiences to nursing theory and practice by reading about the types of patients you care for on your unit. Linking theory to practice as you visualize the patients you've cared for, including their symptoms, assessment data, lab values, etc., will help build your critical thinking skills.

You've already developed strong reading habits in nursing school – you couldn't have survived without this skill. Continue those good reading habits throughout your career. Start with the most frequently seen diagnoses on your unit. Also read about common treatments, medications and procedures for these conditions.

Read professional journals, including a general nursing journal such as *American Journal of Nursing (AJN)*, *RN Magazine* or *Nursing*. Also read a journal related to your specialized area of nursing. This habit will not only help you grow as a nurse, but will also keep you abreast of the latest developments in nursing and evidence-based care.

Observe Procedures

As much as possible, observe procedures that are performed on the patients most typically cared for on your unit, such as surgeries, cardiac catheterizations, Cesarean sections, PICC line insertions, bronchoscopies and other procedures as appropriate. This will help you in many ways, including:

• Building empathy as you witness the patient's experience.

• Enhancing patient teaching – you'll be better able to teach your patients about what to expect after seeing the procedures firsthand.

• Increasing your general knowledge about patient care on your unit.

Hopefully, observing the procedures typical on your unit is a built-in component of your orientation experience. If not, talk to your preceptor and if necessary, your supervisor or manager to make sure this can be part of your orientation plan.

Practice Procedures to Build Skills and Confidence

As a new RN, you're building both your knowledge base and your technical skill level. When you were in nursing school, you learned and performed many technical skills. But as you launch your new career, there are probably some skills you either didn't get the opportunity to perform on a "live" patient, or you need more practice to build competency.

During our careers, your authors have seen new RNs shy away from procedures they're uncomfortable with, such as starting IVs or inserting NG tubes and Foley catheters, only to find themselves struggling with these skills when they're off orientation and don't have a resource nurse readily available to help them.

Don't avoid practicing these skills and procedures, especially during your new graduate orientation or residency program, when you can perform them with your preceptor.

Look for opportunities to build your skills. For example, if you're uncomfortable with IV starts, ask other team members to alert you when they have an IV insertion to perform. Have your preceptor or another nurse coach you through the procedure. Do this as often as needed to build your comfort and confidence with the skill.

"Knowledge is power! As I felt my knowledge grow, I felt more confident with myself and I was able to project that confidence in my daily assignments and interactions with patients and their loved ones." Lourdes Salandanan

Read Lourdes' story, *Building Your Competence While Growing Your Confidence,* on page 232.

Attend Continuing Education Courses

As part of your new grad or residency program, you'll probably attend courses about general nursing care, hospital policies and procedures and education related specifically to your nursing department.

As you progress in your development as an RN, attend classes to further expand your knowledge. Many organizations offer continuing education courses for staff. As an employee, you may also have the benefit of paid continuing education hours. Explore your options and take advantage of them.

Nursing Grand Rounds

During the past few years, there has been a resurgence of nursing grand rounds in many hospitals. Nursing grand rounds focus specifically on nursing's interventions and contributions to the care of the patient. Nursing staff and clinical experts present case studies, discuss best practices, examine new care modalities and share data on nurse-sensitive outcomes in a learning environment that encourages professional debate and inquiry.

Nursing grand rounds provide a dynamic learning experience directed at improving practice and quality of patient care. This forum provides new RNs with the opportunity to observe senior nurses and nurse experts discussing elements of professional nursing practice and integrating nursing's unique contributions to the overall plan of patient care.

Always Seek Opportunities to Learn and Grow

Although you've recently finished school, your learning has just begun. Nursing is a profession that promotes lifelong learning. Seek every opportunity to learn and grow by attending classes, observing procedures, asking questions and reading to expand knowledge. These habits you establish early in your career will be crucial as you evolve from novice to expert.

Building Your Professional Toolkit Through Education

Brenda shares this story:

I was receiving report on my patients in preparation for the 12-hour night shift on my cardiac telemetry unit. Mrs. *T* was a post-heart catheterization patient from another hospital. The heart cath showed coronary artery blockages and she was scheduled for stent placement the next day. During report, the day shift nurse related that Mrs. *T* was "a little uncomfortable" and her blood pressure had "dropped a little" over the past hour.

When I entered Mrs. *T*'s room, she looked uncomfortable and was complaining of lower back pain. Over the past two hours, her BP had steadily dropped from 124/80 to the current reading of 96/64. I followed our standardized procedure for low blood pressure and started a 500 cc bolus of normal saline, then paged her cardiologist. The cardiologist said that the IV bolus should bring up her blood pressure. When her blood pressure was higher, I was to administer IV Morphine for her back pain.

But Mrs. *T*'s BP didn't rise, and instead continued to drop slowly. Her back pain was growing more severe and she also felt an overwhelming urge to have a bowel movement. Just the week before, I had attended a lecture by a cardiologist about complications from interventional procedures. Mrs. *T* was exhibiting all the symptoms he described of a retro-peritoneal bleed – a very rare complication resulting from accessing the femoral artery for the heart cath. I called her cardiologist twice more. He was becoming increasingly annoyed with my calls and gave no orders. I told him that if he didn't come to the unit and examine Mrs. *T*, I would call our department's medical director.

I asked some of the veteran nurses for advice, and they had no additional suggestions beyond what I had already done. When I mentioned retro-peritoneal bleed, one said: "That's so rare; we've never even had a patient with a bleed like that on this floor. That can't be the problem."

Before I could call the medical director, Mrs. *T*'s cardiologist arrived on the unit. He took one look at Mrs. *T* and the record of her blood pressure readings for the past few hours and was very concerned, yet puzzled, as to what the problem could be. He asked me if I had any ideas, and I again relayed the information I had learned in the recent lecture I attended about retro-peritoneal bleeds. "That hardly ever happens," he replied. "Let's try to come up with something a little more realistic."

He ordered Mrs. *T*'s immediate transfer to the ICU. I had already alerted the house supervisor about the patient's condition and there was an ICU bed waiting for her. The cardiologist paged one of his senior partners to meet him in the ICU. I got someone to help me, and we transferred the patient. When I got back to our unit, the senior cardiologist was on the phone requesting to speak to me. "I hear you think this patient has a retro-peritoneal bleed," he said. I braced myself for some negative comments, but instead he said: "I don't know how you knew it, but you're right. We're sending her to surgery for a repair. I wish someone would have listened to you sooner!"

This experience taught me that we continue to grow our skills and knowledge as RNs through many experiences, both on the job and in a classroom setting. The key is applying this knowledge when caring for our patients.

Questions for Reflection

1. As a newly licensed RN, you're in Patricia Benner's novice stage of development. What are the characteristics of this stage?

2. What are some strategies you can utilize to move to the next stage?

3. Think about your preceptor or another RN on your unit. Which of Benner's stages of development are they in? What are the characteristics of this stage?

4. Describe an interaction or situation in which you made a positive contribution to a patient's outcome. This could be a situation where you acted independently or with others on the team. How did helping this patient make you feel?

Paving the Road:
Preceptors, Mentors and Role Models

"People never improve unless they look to some standard or example higher and better than themselves."
Tyron Edwards

As we discussed in Chapter 1, successfully moving through the stages of novice to expert will depend mainly on your commitment, motivation, willingness to learn and perseverance through difficult situations. But you don't have to go it alone. Although this is your journey, there will be many people along the way to guide, influence and support you.

They are preceptors, mentors and role models. They play key roles in helping you attain success – not just as a new nurse – but throughout your career.

Your Preceptor

As a new graduate nurse, you'll participate in some type of on-the-job training program. Depending on your employer, this can range from formal residencies with structured training and experiences founded on evidence-based learning strategies to more informal training where your experiences are directed mainly by you and your preceptor.

Regardless of the program, most include a combination of simulation, didactic or classroom training, experiences that will enhance your knowledge of the type of patients you'll be caring for, orientation to your new organization and on-the-job precepted training on the unit where you'll be working.

"One of the richest blessings in my nursing career has been Maureen, my first preceptor as a new graduate..." Debra Brady

Read Debra's story, *The Blessing of My Preceptor*, on page 226.

For example: Carol was just hired for a cardiac telemetry unit. Her 16-week "new graduate program" will include new employee and hospital orientation classes; classroom presentations on patient safety, time management, delegation, communication skills and other general topics that all new grads in the organization will attend; and observation of cardiac procedures such as heart catheterization and coronary artery bypass surgery. Carol will spend the remainder of her 16-week program working on her new unit under the guidance of a clinical preceptor.

In those early days as a new nurse, your preceptor is one of the most important people to guide you on your journey. Your preceptor is your primary resource and a role model as you learn the daily routines and what's expected of a nurse on your new unit. Your preceptor will guide, coach and teach you for a specified period of time. In many programs, the two of you will share one assignment. You'll gradually assume increasing levels of responsibility until you're able to care for the entire patient assignment.

Your preceptor is usually not the most senior or expert nurse on the unit. As we discussed in the previous chapter, expert nurses practice at such a high level, it may be difficult for them to train you at the novice stage. Instead, the RNs who have the skills and knowledge to successfully care for the patients on the unit, yet are still familiar with the issues faced by a new grad, often make ideal preceptors.

In many organizations, preceptors complete a course or training program to help them in this role. Although preceptors are usually assigned to their orientees by the manager, these RNs usually volunteer for this role. Maybe they enjoy teaching. Perhaps they want to ensure that new nurses on their unit are successful – so they play an active role in making this happen. Or maybe they had a positive experience with their own preceptor, and want to give back to the profession by helping you. No matter what the reason, be comforted in knowing that your preceptor probably chose this role. Although precepting a new nurse at times can be stressful and more work, don't ever feel you're a burden to your preceptor. Remember, your preceptor most likely volunteered for this role.

Good Communication is Key to a Positive Relationship with Your Preceptor

As you work with your preceptor, keep in mind that good communication is critical to a successful relationship. Initially, your preceptor will be doing much of the talking as they instruct you on the workings of the unit and the care of patients. But as you become more comfortable, the dialogue should evolve to two-way communication where you discuss patient care, unit culture, interactions with physicians, etc. Don't be hesitant to ask questions or express any needs you have. This is your time to learn, and you're working with an experienced nurse whose goal is to help you learn and grow. Develop strategies with your preceptor to build your knowledge and skills and optimize this valuable time together.

As you'll soon learn, patient care and day-to-day tasks on the unit will keep you and your preceptor very busy. However, it's important to find time to set goals, discuss your progress, assess and re-prioritize your needs, and redefine the orientation plan as needed. Sometimes, you may even need to meet off-shift to discuss your training. Some organizations or units will set times for preceptor-preceptee meetings, others may expect these meetings to be done during the shift. Whatever the process, meeting regularly with your preceptor is a must.

Most organizations have checklists or guidelines to help you and your preceptor develop a plan and track your progress. If there is no formal checklist or guidelines for new graduates or the existing guidelines seem inadequate, then work with your preceptor to develop a plan. For example, if there is one overall checklist for your orientation, then work with your preceptor to develop daily and weekly goals.

Review and evaluate your progress each shift. This is especially important when you work 12-hour shifts – you work fewer days each week and have so much learning and information packed into each day. Touching bases at the end of the shift and briefly planning for the next one will help you stay on track and get the most from your training experience.

As you meet with your preceptor, celebrate what you've accomplished and develop plans to fill in the gaps. Be honest in communicating your needs. For example:

"I noticed we have a small but steady number of total hip replacement patients on the unit. I've only cared for one so far, and I'm still feeling uncomfortable with their post-op care and how to position and move them. Can we request one of these patients on our next shift?"

Your preceptor will then work with the charge nurse to ensure you're assigned the patients and experiences you need to make the most of your orientation. But without this two-way dialogue, your preceptor won't be able to accurately gauge your comfort level with different types of patients and situations.

What if I'm Not Getting Along with My Preceptor?

Even though your new manager tries to match you with a preceptor who will be a good fit, sometimes the relationship can be problematic. Perhaps you and your preceptor have differing values. Maybe your communication styles or personalities are so different that you're having trouble relating to each other. Or it could be your preceptor thought they'd enjoy teaching, only to find they're very uncomfortable with it.

Whatever the reason, you have to deal with it in order to maximize your learning and successfully transition to your new role as a nurse. Here are some basic steps you can take to rectify the situation:

Assess your situation. What's working well? What are your issues and needs? If you have problems and/or needs that aren't being met, honestly determine the cause. Is it related to your preceptor and their expectations? Your knowledge and/or skill level? Circumstances beyond anyone's control? A combination of several factors? Or are you expecting too much from yourself as a new graduate?

Communicate your issues and needs to your preceptor. In chapters 4 and 5 we go into great detail about effective communication in difficult situations. Review those chapters for strategies to help you frame this potentially sensitive conversation. When communicating with your preceptor, be sure to listen to their perspective. Understanding their viewpoint will hopefully address some or all of your concerns and/or help the two of you make adjustments to rectify the situation. Discuss and compare your expectations with your preceptor's. Are they similar or very different? Redefining goals and expectations may be necessary.

If you believe that talking with your preceptor about these issues would make the situation worse, start with a small concern and see how your preceptor responds. If the conversation goes well, then you can move on to other things. If the conversation doesn't go well, then you may need to enlist help from a third party. But only after you've attempted to resolve the situation with your preceptor.

Talk with a third party about your issues. If your health care organization has a formal residency or new graduate program, there's probably an RN, often a nurse educator or clinical nurse specialist, who oversees the orientation program. This would be a good person to speak to about your issue. This nurse can often provide you with valuable advice, or may even mediate a discussion between you and your preceptor. Depending on the situation, they may discuss the issue with your unit manager. Make sure they gain your permission before taking this step. If there is no such person designated in your organization, seek advice from an experienced nurse you trust.

"Speak up for yourself when things aren't working!"
Jennifer Friedenbach

Read Jennifer's story, *Even New Grads Can Take Charge*, on page 239.

Speak with your manager. If there's is no third party or this option didn't provide a satisfactory solution, then speak with your unit manager about the issue. They will strive to come up with a solution to help you be successful – whether it be giving you advice, mediating a conversation with your preceptor, taking a more active role in your orientation or assigning you to a new preceptor.

But remember, before speaking to your manager, try your other options. One of the first questions they may ask you is: "What have you done so far to solve the problem?"

Orientation Red Flags and Possible Solutions

• You're assigned multiple preceptors with little or no continuity in the messages you receive from each of them.

What to do: Request to be assigned just one preceptor. Be willing to change your schedule to match your preceptor's. If part of the problem is that the "really good teachers" on your new unit all work part-time, then having two preceptors would be beneficial. Request that the three of you meet periodically to discuss your goals and progress so that everyone is on the same page.

Some organizations have an effective orientation system where multiple preceptors are utilized, each with expertise in a specific area or system, such as pulmonary, cardiac, neurology, etc. This type of orientation can be very beneficial as long as the underlying messages delivered by each preceptor don't conflict.

• There are very few guidelines about what is expected of you and/or the time frames to meet these objectives.

What to do: Ask for a meeting with your manager and preceptor to set these objectives and time frames. Discuss your performance and needs daily with your preceptor. Perhaps the documents you use can be modified as needed and used by unit staff for orientation of other new grad RNs.

• You don't feel your preceptor is listening to your concerns and suggestions about your orientation.

What to do: Set a time to discuss your orientation with your preceptor. Ideally, a time can be selected that's not during your shift so the two of you aren't distracted with patient care duties. Be focused and direct with your preceptor about your concerns. Ask your preceptor to describe their preferred communication style – perhaps part of the problem is that the two of you have very different ways of communicating. Agree on strategies for improving your communication to each other. When you're back on the floor, if your preceptor isn't sticking to these agreed-upon strategies, remind them of what you discussed.

• You and your preceptor frequently have more patients than a regular assignment for one nurse. You're told this is acceptable because "there are two of you."

What to do: Hopefully, your preceptor will intervene with the manager/charge nurse to make sure this only happens in emergency situations. If that doesn't work, the two of you should speak to your unit manager about this issue.

Mentors

Unlike preceptors who are appointed to be teachers and coaches for a limited time period, a mentor is someone experienced in a specific area you're interested in. A mentor helps you grow personally and professionally in a safe environment through advice, guidance and pushing you to reach your potential. There is no set time period for this relationship.

Dictionary.com defines mentor as a "wise and trusted counselor or teacher; an influential senior sponsor or supporter." The term mentor originated thousands of years ago in Homer's book, *The Odyssey*. The character, Mentor, was a loyal and valued advisor to King Odysseus, and he was also entrusted with the education of Odysseus' son. Throughout history, mentors have helped guide their mentees to achieve their full potential.

Some famous mentor-mentee relationships you may recognize:

Alexander the Great, mentored by Aristotle
Mozart, mentored by Johann Bach
Helen Keller, mentored by Anne Sullivan
Luke Skywalker, mentored by Yoda and Obi-Wan Kenobi
Harry Potter, mentored by Professor Albus Dumbledore

Although many professions have formal mentor programs where mentors are assigned to proteges, in nursing this relationship is often more informal with an experienced nurse taking another nurse "under their wing." The more experienced nurse recognizes the mentee's potential and helps them grow, through advice, support and constructive feedback.

Shelia Grossman, author of *Mentoring in Nursing: A Dynamic and Collaborative Process*, defines mentoring as:

"...a guided experience, formally or informally assigned, that empowers the mentor and mentee to develop personally and professionally within the auspices of a caring, collaborative, culturally competent and respected environment."

A mentor is not someone who will accomplish a goal for you, but instead will show you how to achieve the goal for yourself. A mentor provides a safe haven for you to share ideas, vent your frustrations, problem-solve solutions and receive honest feedback in a nonthreatening manner.

Most successful nurses have had mentors at various stages of their careers. For some nurses, their first mentor was their preceptor, who continued to guide and support them after their formal preceptor relationship ended. Later, they identified other mentors to help them in their chosen paths, for example: moving from med/surg to critical care, leaving acute care nursing to join academia or choosing to pursue a career in management.

There is no limit to the number of mentors who may positively influence you professionally and personally. And mentors don't always need to be RNs. They are people with expertise in areas you'd like to learn more about.

"When I look back at my first year of nursing, I know that I wouldn't have survived without Rosemary. She held me up, pumped me full of confidence and with her as a mirror, I developed a 'can-do' attitude." Kay Evans

Read Kay's story, *Finding Your Lifeline*, on page 230.

Mentors See Our Potential

Pat shares this story:

My siblings and I were the first generation in our family to attend college. Conversations around our dinner table were never about if you would go to college, but rather which school you would attend. When I was accepted to the local associate degree nursing program, my parents were delighted. My father had been a corpsman in the Army and held registered nurses in the highest esteem.

We were fortunate that my uncle, who never married, gave each of us kids US Saving Bonds three to four times a year throughout our childhood. His generosity covered my college tuition and books. He was much older than my father and developed congestive heart failure when he was in his early 70s. His condition continued to deteriorate resulting in repeated hospitalizations. He became a regular patient at the community hospital where I worked as an RN. My father would visit him daily, and unbeknownst to me, our director and associate director of nursing would visit them during their rounds. Apparently, the conversations would focus on the importance of education, specifically my education.

My two mentors had been encouraging me to return to school. I was planning to get a bachelor's degree in health administration and later become a pediatric nurse practitioner, a path that was embraced by many nurses in the early 1980s. However, this wasn't the path my mentors envisioned for me.

When my uncle passed away, my father told me he had made arrangements in his will for me to return to school. However the caveat was that I must attend the University of California, San Francisco to earn both a BSN and MSN, which I did.

My mentors saw my potential – they believed in me and encouraged me throughout my time at UCSF. I remained connected to these two women throughout my career. Unfortunately, they both passed away far too soon. Today, even as a veteran of almost 40 years in practice, I think about the advice they gave me – it's as relevant today as it was when I first received it.

My recommendation for new nurses is to find a mentor – you and your career will flourish!

How Do I Choose a Mentor?

"The strongest relationships spring out of a real and often earned connection felt by both sides." Sheryl Sandberg

• Identify colleagues who excel in areas you're interested in and are willing to help you build your skills. This could be an RN who performs exemplary patient care. Maybe someone who is well-versed in evidence-based practice and quality improvement. Or perhaps you want to improve your communication skills and you identify a colleague with excellent abilities in this area.

In addition to the subject they excel in, also pay attention to their interpersonal skills, values and work ethic. Do they have a positive attitude? Are they good team players and interact positively with colleagues? You don't want a mentor who doesn't share your values or will teach you bad habits. You want mentors to challenge you to reach your potential.

• Start to build a relationship with that person. Ask them questions. Seek their guidance. Are they open to helping you and teaching you?

• If yes, then tell them you respect and admire their skills in their area of excellence. Ask if they will mentor you in this area.

• Have realistic expectations of what you want your mentor to help you with. Communicate these expectations to your mentor. What are their expectations?

• Set realistic goals together. Periodically review the goals. Revise goals as needed.

• Be willing to accept and give honest feedback.

In some cases, mentors will find you and initiate the relationship. This can happen for a variety of reasons, but it's often because these individuals were helped and mentored by others and want to give back to the profession by taking a colleague under their wing.

Not every nurse has or wants a mentor. Except in rare instances when a mentor is assigned to you, it will be up to you to choose one. Your authors highly recommend mentor relationships. We've both grown personally and professionally through our relationships with mentors at various stages of our careers and probably would not be in our current positions if not for our mentors. We wish the same success for you!

"It's important to look for those colleagues who are willing to help you be successful." Alison Riggs

Read Alison's story, My Almost First Nursing Job, on page 268.

Role Models

According to *Dictionary.com*, a role model is someone whose "behavior, actions or success is emulated by others." In some cases, we may not have a relationship with, or even personally know the role model. It's common for teenagers to look up to celebrities and sports figures as their role models. Many nurses will tell you Florence Nightingale is one of their role models.

We can have role models for various aspects of our lives – personal, professional, community service and even sports. As teenagers in the 1970s, your authors along with many other teenaged female tennis players, adopted the two-handed backhand, just like our role model – tennis star Chris Evert, who made this tennis stroke famous. Today, many teenage girls who play tennis try to mimic the near-perfect play of Serena Williams.

Role models are important because they provide us with a standard to emulate and strive for. As a new graduate nurse, some of your early nursing role models were probably your nursing faculty and the nurses you observed in your clinical rotations. As you launch your nursing career, your first role model in your new job is often your preceptor. As you observe other nurses, you'll likely expand your list of role models.

There is no perfect nurse who possesses all the right qualities. Instead, you'll probably have different role models for different areas of your nursing practice. One or more nurses may be role models for exceptional patient care. Another may be your role model for exemplary communication and leadership skills.

Brenda's Role Models:

My mother – My role model for living a positive life.

Leah Curtin, nurse, writer, editor and ethicist – Although I've never met her, Leah showed me that you can build a fulfilling career as both a nurse and a writer.

Patricia McFarland – My co-author, who exemplifies visionary leadership. After nearly 40 years as an RN, Pat continues to be a passionate advocate for the nursing profession and quality patient care.

Barbara – My unit's day shift charge nurse was my first role model as a new graduate. She was an expert nurse, who was knowledgeable, patient, compassionate and kept a cool head in emergencies. Her sense of humor helped alleviate many tense and stressful situations. She later became a mentor to me.

Pat's Role Models:

My grandmother – She lived to be 102 years old. Despite having only a fourth grade education, she was articulate, well-read and was a talented seamstress who was always impeccably dressed. Her humor and ability to laugh at herself are traits I try to emulate.

Nish – A nurse who cared for me when I was hospitalized as a child. I set the goal of becoming a nurse after that hospital stay. I later worked with Nish and she became a mentor to me.

My father – His strong ethics and passion for life were an inspiration to me.

My mother – Her commitment to reading and learning set the example for me to pursue lifelong learning.

Who are your role models?

Building Your Support System

Preceptors, mentors and role models. Very important people who help you develop into the best nurse possible. But even though they're outstanding in their practice or area of expertise – they're not perfect. If you observe them long enough, you'll notice they have their own mentors and role models to help them expand their knowledge and expertise. Because no matter how skilled, knowledgeable or experienced any of us are – no one has all the answers!

Strive to reach your full potential, celebrate your achievements and create a support system to help you continue to learn and grow.

Questions for Reflection

1. Make a list of the skills and competencies you feel you need to develop. Discuss this list with your preceptor and come up with a plan to build your experience in these areas.

2. You're in the 6th week of your 16-week residency program. You would like to take on more responsibility for the patient assignment, but your preceptor is telling you to wait until you have more experience. What should you do?

3. You feel that your preceptor is not very available to help you. When you look for her, she's often in the staff lounge or off the unit. What should you do?

4. You've noticed that your preceptor cuts corners and doesn't always follow the standards of care. What should you do?

5. You're coming to the end of your preceptorship and you feel that you could use another week. Who do you talk to about this? How would you frame the conversation?

Defining Your Role as an RN: Important Resources to Guide Your Practice

"The most important practical lesson that can be given to nurses is to teach them what to observe."

Florence Nightingale

Through your academic preparation you were exposed to the art and science of nursing practice. Now as a newly licensed RN, you're ready to begin practicing. Are you prepared to embrace the true essence of professional nursing?

A wise mentor once said that the first two years of practice are the most important in a nurse's career. During our first years of practice, we're socialized as professionals and begin to truly understand what it means to be registered nurses. Initially most new graduates are focused on skill acquisition, rather than role transition. Although acquiring the skills necessary to care for patients is extremely important, socialization as a professional nurse is critical for overall success in the profession.

Regardless of whether you're launching your career in a formal residency program or practicing under the watchful eye of an experienced nurse, you'll be exposed to resources and tools that will assist you in your transition.

Just as every building needs a solid foundation if it's to stand the test of time, our nursing careers must be built on a strong foundation. The foundation of nursing practice is our professional scope of practice, standards of practice and code of ethics. Our state-specific nurse practice acts, including their accompanying rules and regulations, are superimposed over our professional standards and ethics. Hospital and institutional policies and procedures integrate aspects of our scope, standards and practice act.

Our purpose with this chapter is to introduce you to several valuable resources that will help you build a solid foundation for nursing practice. Like carpenters, who add tools to their toolkits as they perfect their craft, you too will begin to add resources and tools to your professional nursing toolkit. Your toolkit will range from professional documents to favorite websites. Over the course of your career, you'll find that you refer to these resources time and time again.

Many of these same tools are used by nurse leaders as they evaluate nursing practice, develop policies and implement system changes to drive improvements in patient care. Having an understanding and appreciation of their importance is your first step toward professionalism. Your preceptors and mentors will offer additional tools, but for our discussion let's focus on the following items:

- Characteristics of a professional
- American Nurses Association's (ANA) *Nursing's Social Policy Statement*
- Your personal definition of nursing
- The nursing process
- ANA *Scope and Standards of Practice*
- ANA *Code of Ethics for Nurses*
- *Nurse Practice Act* for the state in which you're licensed and practicing

In addition, you'll find the following items very important for your success:

- An understanding of the standards of practice for your specialty. For example, if you are a critical care RN, you would also be expected to have an understanding of the American Association of Critical Care Nurses' (AACN) *Standards of Practice*. The AACN standards delineate expectations for practitioners working in the critical care arena. Nurses working in women's health should be familiar with the standards published by their national organization, Association of Women's Health, Obstetric and Neonatal Nurses (AWHONN). Both of these national associations use the ANA standards as the framework for their standards development.

- Your employer's (hospital, health system, clinic, etc.) specific policies, procedures and protocols related to your practice.

- Your current job description and the job descriptions of those you supervise.

"Each day as you go into your workplace, never forget the huge responsibility of your role as an RN." Kimberly Horton

Read Kimberly's story, *What Being a Nurse is Really About*, on page 182.

Suggested websites to include in your toolkit:

- Board of Nursing for the state in which you're licensed and practicing. Or if you're part of the multi-state compact, your "home" state and the state in which you practice (we'll discuss the multi-state compact later in this chapter).
- National Council of State Boards of Nursing (www.ncsbn.com).
- American Nurses Association (www.nursingworld.com).
- Your specialty organization.

Nursing as a Profession

For decades we've debated the question: *Is nursing a profession?* Nursing has struggled with its identity as a profession for many years. Some believe that the multiple avenues to RN licensure is at the core of this struggle. Nurses continue to debate the issue while other health care disciplines have elevated their educational requirements for licensure to the clinical doctorate. Over the past several years, we've seen a growing body of evidence providing a positive correlation between a better educated nursing workforce and improved patient outcomes.

In 2010, the Institute of Medicine issued the ground-breaking report, *The Future of Nursing: Leading Change, Advancing Health.* In this report, the IOM recommends that nurse leaders in academia and service work collaboratively with regulators and policy-makers to streamline the education process so that by 2020, 80 percent of registered nurses are prepared at the baccalaureate level.

Nursing educators across the country have been collaborating to streamline the educational process making it easier for nurses to continue their education. At this point, we are not saying that entry into our profession must be at the baccalaureate level. However, we are clearly saying that nursing, like all professions, requires a commitment to lifelong learning and the utilization of evidence to improve practice.

Webster.com defines a profession as "an occupation that requires extensive education or training, the purpose of which is to supply objective counsel and service to others." Based on our experience and review of the literature, we would like to add that a profession is also based on a theoretical and evidence-based foundation, where members embrace lifelong learning to further advancements within the profession.

The literature contains numerous descriptions of behaviors and attributes of professionals. Simply type the word "profession" or "professional" into a search engine and numerous definitions appear. We've compiled a list of the most common professional behaviors and characteristics appearing in the literature.

While reviewing the list, contemplate each of these behaviors. As a newly licensed nurse, consider how you will embrace these characteristics:

- Professionals have specialized knowledge acquired through extensive formal education.

- Professionals embrace and are committed to lifelong learning.

- Professionals accept personal responsibility for their actions and practice.

- Professionals take pride and ownership in their work.

- Professionals understand the importance of relationships and collaboration with peers, colleagues and members of the team.

- Professionals commit to and maintain personal and professional integrity and ethics.

- Professionals strive for excellence in their practice.

Dr. Maria O'Rourke, a leading authority on professional practice, reminds us that nurses, like all members of the health care team, must embrace the professional role and its associated obligations. The common thread among members of the health care team is the fact that we're all professionals. Therefore, each member of the team can be held to these same standards. It is through our discipline-specific scope and standards of practice that we begin to articulate and integrate our contributions to the care of the patient, family and community. As you grow in your RN role, you'll integrate these behaviors into your practice. When we understand and appreciate the fact that all health care disciplines are professionals first, our conversations have the potential to change dramatically. It's only when we fail to show up as professionals that our position on the interdisciplinary team is at risk of being devalued.

Later in this chapter, we'll discuss the ANA *Code of Ethics*. It will then become clearer how these characteristics are interwoven into our professional standards and ethics.

Defining Nursing

Patients are admitted to the hospital for nursing care! Nursing is the profession that's with the patient 24 hours a day, 7 days a week. We are the discipline welcomed into the homes of our frail elderly, home bound and hospice clients. Nursing's plan of care includes moving the patient to their optimal level of health or to a peaceful death. RNs are responsible for bringing nursing's unique contribution to the interdisciplinary team discussion.

At this point in your career, you may still be struggling with your personal definition of nursing. The definition of nursing has evolved since the early days of Florence Nightingale, the founder of modern nursing. In her book, *Notes on Nursing*, Nightingale wrote: "What nursing has to do is to put the patient in the best condition for nature to act upon him." While this definition appears simplistic, don't forget it was Nightingale who recognized the importance of evidence to drive nursing practice. Today, the American Nurses Association (ANA) defines nursing as:

"The protection, promotion, and optimization of health and abilities, prevention of illness and injury, alleviation of suffering through the diagnosis and treatment of human responses, and advocacy in the care of individuals, families, communities and populations."

This definition, or one very similar, is most likely what your faculty used as a foundation to begin your nursing education. In reality, organizations, schools, employers and individuals may put slightly different spins on the ANA definition in an effort to tailor it to the institution or organization.

Over the years, your authors have found that our definitions of nursing and nursing practice have evolved. Our roles, education and experiences in nursing have shaped our personal definitions of what nursing is and is not.

We encourage you to take a few minutes to write your personal definition of nursing. Put your definition in an envelope and seal it. On the first anniversary of receiving your license, open the envelope and read what you wrote. You'll be amazed to see how your personal definition evolved. In one short year, you'll begin to see nursing practice in a very different light based on your experiences and socialization to the profession. Continue to do this each year to re-energize your passion for nursing.

"While studying nursing, I never realized the impact I could make in people's lives by being a nurse." Julian Gallegos

Read Julian's story, *Caring for My Wounded Brothers and Sisters,* **on page 214.**

Social Policy, Scope and Standards of Practice, and Code of Ethics

As professionals, we look to ANA as the organization responsible for the protection, promotion and advancement of nursing practice. For more than 100 years, ANA has been the professional organization that sets and defines our scope and standards of practice.

To help us understand the depth and breadth of nursing practice, ANA has published three books which build upon nursing's unique accountability to society, while describing the essence of nursing through definitions and standards. These three books: *Nursing's Social Policy Statement, Scope and Standards of Practice,* and *Code of Ethics for Nurses,* will be your lifeline to professional practice throughout your career. Let's briefly look at each of these documents to help you understand why we believe they are critical in helping you build a solid professional practice foundation.

Even after many years in the nursing profession, your authors continue to use these resources. Every nurse's library should include these documents either in hard copy or as part of your e-library. The three publications can be purchased independently or as a set from the ANA website at www.nursingworld.com.

Here is a brief description of these valuable resources from ANA:

Nursing's Social Policy Statement: The Essence of the Profession

"Nursing is the pivotal health care profession, highly valued for its specialized knowledge, skill, and caring in improving the health status of the public and ensuring safe, effective, quality care." ANA

The ANA social policy statement serves as a resource to assist nurses in conceptualizing professional practice. This document gives direction to educators, administrators and researchers as they further the work of nursing. The statement informs not only the profession but also the public about nursing's social responsibility, accountability and contributions to the health of our communities. From this document, we begin to understand the definition of nursing, as well as the purpose of the scope and standards of nursing practice.

The Nursing Process

The nursing process is the RN's critical thinking model. Our professional standards and practice acts are grounded in the nursing process. The nursing process is one of the most important tools newly licensed RNs can utilize, not only to transition to your new role as a practicing nurse, but to use throughout your career.

As a reminder, the steps of the nursing process are:

- Assessment
- Diagnosis
- Outcomes identification
- Planning
- Implementation
- Evaluation

It's important to remember that the nursing process is not a linear model, but rather a dynamic process that's in continuous motion, resulting in constant assessment and re-assessment.

Your ability to analyze data from multiple sources, integrate your assessment and findings into a nursing diagnosis, and as a result, implement a patient-specific plan of care, becomes second nature as you gain experience, confidence and competence. Too frequently, newly licensed RNs forget the final step in the nursing process – evaluation. Never underestimate the power of utilizing all the steps in the nursing process. Evaluating the patient's response to your actions and interventions is as critical to the process as completing a comprehensive assessment.

Nursing: Scope and Standards of Practice

This document clarifies the RN's scope of practice by framing the professional role of nurses in the United States. The ANA *Scope of Practice* statement essentially answers the who, what, when, where, why and how of nursing practice. These standards apply to all practicing RNs. Through these standards, we further define our responsibilities and accountabilities to our profession, patients and society. As you become more confident and competent, you'll want to participate in the continuous development and review of these standards through collaboration with peers and participation in a professional organization such as ANA. It is through the ongoing refinement and development of our standards of practice that nursing care remains relevant and based on current evidence.

Standards of Professional Practice are the authoritative statements of the duties that all RNs, regardless of role, population or specialty, are expected to perform competently. Our values and priorities as a profession are reflected in these standards. The *Standards of Professional Nursing Practice* can be divided into two sections: *Standards of Practice* and *Standards of Professional Performance*. The six *Standards of Practice* are actually the identified steps in the nursing process. As we stated earlier, the nursing process is the adopted critical thinking model utilized by nursing professionals, while the ten standards of professional performance identify competent behaviors of the professional nurse.

The primary purpose for nursing competence is to protect the public. As professionals we're also committed to maintaining competence to ensure the integrity of our profession and advance professional development. It's important to remember that we're all responsible for our own competence. Regulatory agencies set minimal standards for regulating nursing practice, while employers are responsible for creating an environment supporting competent practice. We create synergy when we work together to ensure competence and excellence in patient care.

The table below outlines ANA's *Standards of Practice* and *Standards of Professional Performance*. Although we've listed the ANA *Standards of Practice* for your review, the complete document identifies the specific competencies for each of the standards, for both RNs and advanced practice nurses.

Standards of Professional Nursing Practice

Standards of Practice

Standard 1. Assessment
The registered nurse collects comprehensive data pertinent to the health care consumer's health and/or the situation.

Standard 2. Diagnosis
The registered nurse analyzes the assessment data to determine the diagnosis or the issues.

Standard 3. Outcomes Identification
The registered nurse identifies expected outcomes for a plan individualized to health care consumers or the situation.

Standard 4. Planning
The registered nurse develops a plan that prescribes strategies and alternatives to attain expected outcomes.

Standard 5. Implementation
The registered nurse implements the identified plan:
5A. Coordination of care
5B. Teaching and health promotion
5C. Consultation
5D. Prescriptive authority and treatment

Standard 6. Evaluation
The registered nurse evaluates progress toward attainment of outcomes.

Standards of Professional Performance

Standard 7. Ethics
The registered nurse practices ethically.

Standard 8. Education
The registered nurse attains knowledge and competence that reflect current nursing practice.

Standard 9. Evidence-Based Practice and Research
The registered nurse integrates evidence and research findings into practice.

Standard 10. Quality of Practice
The registered nurse contributes to quality nursing practice.

Standard 11. Communication
The registered nurse communicates effectively.

Standard 12. Leadership
The registered nurse demonstrates leadership in professional practice settings and the profession.

Standard 13. Collaboration
The registered nurse collaborates with the healthcare consumer, family, and others in the conduct of nursing practice.

Standard 14. Professional Practice Evaluation
The registered nurse evaluates her or his own nursing practice in relation to professional practice standards, guidelines, relevant statutes, rules and regulations.

Standard 15. Resource Utilization
The registered nurse utilizes appropriate resources to plan and provide nursing services that are safe, effective, and financially responsible.

Standard 16. Environmental Health
The registered nurse practices in an environmentally safe and healthy manner.

Nursing Scope and Standards, 2nd Edition, 2010

"Beyond being able to care for my patients' health, it is a privilege to share in people's lives." Kendra Bartlow

Read Kendra's story, *The Sweetest Profession of All*, on page 257.

Code of Ethics

"The character of the nurse is as important as the knowledge she or he possesses." Carolyn Jarius

Earlier in this chapter, we identified characteristics of professionals that included maintaining personal and professional integrity and ethics. Having a code of ethics is a hallmark of a true profession. The provisions identified in ANA's *Code of Ethics* will help ground you as you assume your role as a professional nurse.

The ANA *Code of Ethics* helps focus our thinking about ethical issues. It will guide your practice and provide a framework to problem-solve issues that may confront you in your practice setting. Our professional code makes our ethical obligations and duties clear. It clarifies for society what they can expect from professional nurses. (See box on page 52 for ANA's ethical provisions).

As a newly licensed RN, you may find yourself in a quandary regarding an ethical issue. If this happens, you have resources to help guide your actions. Our *Code of Ethics* will help frame your thinking so you can communicate your concerns to your preceptor, manager or other members of the health care team. These senior staff members will help you resolve the situation or work with you to take the ethical issue to your hospital's Ethics Committee. Remember, you're not alone – others will help you address your concerns – but it's your responsibility to communicate the issues.

Facing an Ethical Dilemma: Barry's Story

Pat shares this story:

There are patients who touch our lives and leave a permanent mark on our hearts. One patient who touched my heart was Barry, a young man with massive trauma after being hit by a drunk driver while on his way home from a friend's house.

Barry was in our critical care unit for about eight weeks. His family was wonderfully supportive and loving, even though they knew Barry's outlook was grim. They visited every day, decorated his room and selected inspirational lectures and music to help him "find his way back."

Over the course of his hospitalization, Barry received more than 80 units of blood and blood products. He had a tracheostomy, multiple central lines, a gastrostomy tube and was connected to just about every piece of equipment you could imagine. We maintained his blood pressure and kidney perfusion with the aid of IV drip medications. Barry had been to surgery six times. During his eight weeks in the hospital, Barry had become a shell of who he once was, in spite of our best efforts.

We talked at length with his family about what they thought Barry's wishes would be in these circumstances. Because of his age, they had never discussed the specifics, but as a family they believed he wouldn't want to continue in a vegetative state.

One holiday, Barry began bleeding again. The general surgeon wanted to take him back to surgery. As Barry's nurse, I asked the surgeon what he hoped to gain by operating on Barry again. That was the start of one of the most challenging days in my career. I debated the ethics of performing a seventh operation on Barry for several minutes before the surgeon demanded that I call the nursing supervisor.

From there, we called the chief nursing officer, ICU medical director and chief of staff. It was really a great holiday! The surgeon was furious with me. He accused me of over-stepping my bounds and insisted that I be reprimanded. I held my ground, but not my tongue, as I continued to advocate for Barry.

I suggested we invite the family into the conversation. The family joined a conference call with key members of the Ethics Committee. At the end of the call, the surgeon wrote the order to discontinue the IV drips and allow Barry to die. We waited for his sister to arrive from a neighboring city before we began discontinuing the IV medications. My shift was over, but I asked if I could stay with the family. While the surgeon didn't approve, the members of the Ethics Committee encouraged it.

I have replayed that day in my mind hundreds of times over the years. While I still cry when I think about it, I know I advocated for the patient, his family and their right to have a voice. I learned from this experience that I had resources – professionals who would help me frame the conversation and arrive at the ethical decision.

Guide to the Code of Ethics for Nurses

Provision 1
The nurse, in all professional relationships, practices with compassion and respect for the inherent dignity, worth and uniqueness of every individual, unrestricted by considerations of social or economic status, personal attributes, or the nature of health problems.

Provision 2
The nurse's primary commitment is to the patient, whether an individual, family, group, or community.

Provision 3
The nurse promotes, advocates for, and strives to protect the health, safety, and rights of the patient.

Provision 4
The nurse is responsible and accountable for individual nursing practice and determines the appropriate delegation of tasks consistent with the nurse's obligation to provide optimum patient care.

Provision 5
The nurse owes the same duties to self as to others, including the responsibility to preserve integrity and safety, to maintain competence, and to continue personal and professional growth.

Provision 6
The nurse participates in establishing, maintaining, and improving health care environments and conditions of employment conducive to the provision of quality health care and consistent with the values of the profession through individual and collective action.

Provision 7
The nurse participates in the advancement of the profession through contributions to practice, education, administration, and knowledge development.

Provision 8
The nurse collaborates with other health professionals and the public in promoting community, national, and international efforts to meet health needs.

Provision 9
The profession of nursing, as represented by associations and their members, is responsible for articulating nursing values, for maintaining the integrity of the profession and its practice, and for shaping social policy.

Guide to the Code of Ethics for Nurses - Interpretation and Application; 2010 Reissue

Maintaining Patient Confidentiality

As a professional RN and member of the health care team, ensuring patient confidentiality is one of your ethical responsibilities. In 1996, Congress passed the *Health Insurance Portability and Accountability Act* (HIPAA) to safeguard patient privacy and confidentiality. HIPAA clearly states that it's the entire health care team's responsibility to maintain the privacy and confidentiality of the patients they serve. Confidentiality and privacy protection extends to written, electronic and verbal communication.

As a new RN, you're excited and enthusiastic about what you're learning and doing. You will be tempted to share your experiences with colleagues, friends and family. We caution you to remember that maintaining patient confidentiality is not only the law, but your professional obligation. This means if you don't have a "need to know," then you can't access a patient's medical record or any other source of personal health information.

If you hear colleagues discussing a patient in the elevator or public area, you have the responsibility to tell them to move to a private place to continue their conversation. Patient care information should never be shared on *Facebook* or any other type of social media. What may seem like a harmless posting, can be considered a breach of confidentiality and may jeopardize your career.

Maintaining the Confidentiality of a Celebrity

Pat shares this story:

As a director of nursing in a community-based hospital, I was visiting the oncology unit one afternoon when a nurse approached me about making arrangements for his patient to have her beloved dog visit. I approved his request with the caveat that they let me know when the dog was on the unit.

The dog visited the next day. Later that evening, the patient asked to see me. This patient had been on the unit numerous times over the past several months. I had never met her personally, but knew this would probably be her final admission. As I was about to enter her room, a staff nurse stopped me and asked if I knew this patient was here under an assumed name. I was taken aback. I had no idea that this patient was actually a celebrity. But until that moment, I didn't have a need to know her true identity.

This staff truly understood their personal obligation to maintain a patient's privacy.

Regulating RN Practice

Newly licensed nurses often use the phrase, "I have to protect my license." In reality, the best way to protect your license is to understand the *Nurse Practice Act* in the state in which you practice and ANA's *Standards of Practice* and *Code of Ethics*. Understanding the *Nurse Practice Act*, along with related regulations and standards, will guide your practice and optimize your communication with team members, patients and families.

The National Council of State Boards of Nursing (NCSBN), a nonprofit organization for all state boards of nursing, provides a forum to promote uniform regulations for nursing practice. NCSBN is also responsible for the oversight of the National Certification Licensing Examination (NCLEX). As you know, before you can practice nursing in the United States, you must successfully pass the NCLEX.

Although RNs take a national exam, nursing practice is actually regulated by the state in which the nurse holds their license. However, there is one exception to this statement. Since the late 1990s, states have had the opportunity to participate in the multi-state licensure compact. The Nurse Licensure Compact (NLC) allows a nurse to hold one license in the state of residence (home state), but practice in other states that participate in the compact. A nurse who holds a multi-state license is subject to each state's practice laws and corresponding regulations.

For example:

Mary and Fred graduated from nursing school in South Dakota. Mary applied for and took the NCLEX in North Dakota, her primary state of residence. North Dakota is a member of the Nurse Licensure Compact. Mary has been offered a position in South Dakota. Because both states are members of the NLC, Mary can practice nursing in South Dakota with her North Dakota multi-state license, as long as she does not change her state of residence. If she declares South Dakota her home state by establishing residence there, she will then need to apply for a South Dakota license.

Fred returned home to California where he took the NCLEX and received a California nursing license. California is not currently part of the NLC. Fred was also offered a position in South Dakota. Before he can practice in South Dakota, Fred will need to apply for a South Dakota nursing license, regardless of whether he establishes residency in South Dakota. As long as Fred and Mary practice in South Dakota, their practice will be regulated by the South Dakota *Nurse Practice Act*.

The NCSBN supports collaboration between and among state boards of nursing. An outcome of this collaboration is the mandate that all state practice acts contain key provisions, including: authority, power and composition of a board of nursing; education program standards, and standards and scope of nursing practice; types of titles and licenses; requirements for licensure, and violations and disciplinary action. While the practice act is individualized at the state level, as an RN and consumer of health care, you're guaranteed that a degree of consistency exists across the country regarding state practice acts.

As a registered nurse, you'll want to visit the NCSBN website (www.ncsbn.com) as well as the website(s) for the board of nursing in the state in which you are licensed and practicing. These sites have valuable information for RNs on the practice of nursing as well as newsletters and documents to inform your practice. For newly licensed nurses, the NCSBN's *Frequently Asked Questions* section will be of particular interest.

Because practice parameters for nursing are established by state legislatures, your authority, accountability and responsibility to practice the art and science of nursing is regulated at the state level. The statutory authority for the enforcement of the *Nurse Practice Act* lies with our individual state boards of nursing. The purpose of nursing boards is to protect the public by regulating nursing practice and enforcing the *Nurse Practice Act.*

In most states, the Board of Nursing governs the practice of both RNs and licensed practical nurses (LPN) or licensed vocational nurses (LVN in California and Texas). Four states, California, Georgia, Louisiana and West Virginia, continue to have two nursing boards, the Board of Registered Nursing (BRN) and the Board of Vocational Nursing or Board of Practical Nursing (BVN/BPN). Understanding the oversight structure for nursing in the state in which you practice is yet another aspect of your socialization and transition into your professional nursing role.

Independent, Dependent and Interdependent Practice

State practice acts can include provisions related to independent, dependent and interdependent practice. More than 10 percent of nurses in the US practice in California, so we'll use this state's practice parameters as an example. Remember, if you're licensed in a state other than California, your state's specific practice act will delineate the authority and parameters of your practice.

Independent Practice

RNs have the authority, responsibility and accountability to assess and implement appropriate protocols and interventions based on our professional judgment and the utilization of the nursing process. Independent practice includes those aspects of care that RNs have the authority to assess and implement. This aspect of our practice doesn't require a physician or advanced practitioner's order.

For instance, oral care and elevating the head of the bed for intubated patients are independent nursing practice functions. These activities are evidence-driven nursing interventions that, when implemented, improve the quality of care for patients. Other examples of independent practice may be found in your facility's protocols for fall and pressure ulcer prevention.

As a newly licensed nurse, discuss opportunities and strategies related to independent practice with your preceptor and supervisor frequently. As you grow more confident in your assessments, your need for validation of independent functions will decrease.

Dependent Practice

Dependent practice requires an order from a physician or advanced practice nurse (APN) prior to implementation. Most medications and diagnostic treatments require written orders from an MD or APN. When implementing these orders, we're obligated to question them if, in our professional judgment as RNs, we believe they're not in the best interest of the patient.

Dependent Nursing Practice: Appropriately Questioning an MD Order

Pat shares this story:

As a new graduate, I worked the night shift. The standard of care required the ED physician to notify the internist on call when a patient needed to be admitted. The receiving RN would review the orders from the ED and call the admitting MD for further orders. On this particular night, I was the receiving RN. Our practice was to have a second RN listen to the physician's verbal orders. The primary RN would repeat back the orders and both RNs would then sign the verbal order sheet.

Because the patient was being admitted during shift report, the p.m. shift charge nurse was the second RN on the phone. The physician rattled off the usual orders and I transcribed them without question until he ordered a Foley catheter. I questioned the physician regarding this order. I reminded him that his patient had frequent UTIs and her last hospitalization resulted in a hospital-acquired UTI. He clearly stated that he wanted a Foley catheter to have an accurate output measurement, so I implemented the order.

The following afternoon, the MD came to see the patient. He complained to the p.m. charge nurse that the "young RN" on the night shift falsified his orders. He didn't know that he was speaking to the second RN on the call. The charge nurse asked him specifically which of the orders were incorrect or "falsified." He identified the Foley catheter order.

As the story was related to me, she calmly pointed to her signature on the chart, reminding him that the "young RN" questioned this order. After some backpedaling, he admitted that he ordered the Foley.

If I hadn't followed hospital policy by including the second RN on the phone, it would have been my word against the MD's. Unfortunately, as a new graduate, I may have been on the losing side of that equation.

This situation taught me the importance of following hospital protocol, reading back physician orders, being prepared with patient care data and using my voice to question an order I perceived as not in the best interest of the patient. While the physician ordered the Foley, it was my professional responsibility to question him based on my obligation to demonstrate and transfer scientific knowledge, and apply the nursing process while considering the unique needs of the patient.

Interdependent Practice

Many states have provisions for interdependent practice through the adoption of specific policies and procedures for advanced practice nurses and direct care RNs.

In California, legislators recognize that overlapping practices exist between and among the health professions. The legal mechanism for RNs and APNs to perform functions which would usually be considered the practice of medicine is through the adoption of standardized procedures. These are procedures developed at the system or facility level and require interdisciplinary collaboration and approval. The process for gaining approval to implement procedures that address overlapping practice depends on your state's nurse practice act. Therefore, you'll want to review the practice act to learn the specific requirements related to interdependent practice.

Prior to implementing a standardized procedure in California, the RN must demonstrate competency to perform the specific procedure. Annual competency validation is often required for procedures. The number and type of approved standardized procedures varies from facility to facility. Because standardized procedures are approved at the facility level, as a new RN, you should discuss standardized procedures appropriate for implementation with your preceptor and manager. In California, only RNs can implement standardized procedures. If you practice in a state other than California, review your state's practice act to determine what is required to implement standardized procedures or delegated medical procedures and who is authorized to practice under them.

Throughout our careers in nursing, your authors have seen changes in practice over time. What may have required a standardized procedure in the past, today may be considered independent practice.

Interdependent Nursing Practice

Pat shares this story:

As director of nursing in a faith-based community hospital, I was responsible for nursing practice in several large inpatient units, as well as a large hospital-based distinct part skilled nursing facility (HBDP/SNF) located across the street from the main campus. Prior to moving the unit across the street, it had been located within the acute care hospital. Practice at that time was to call the emergency department physician when a patient expired. The ED physician would come to the HBDP/SNF and pronounce the patient. Once the HBDP/SNF moved across the street, this was no longer accepted practice.

This presented a unique problem for the nursing staff. We discussed the issue at our nursing council and with our medical director. The solution was to write a standardized procedure enabling an RN to determine when a patient had expired. It was approved by the medical staff and implemented by the registered nurses, not only in the HBDP/SNF, but throughout the hospital. This practice change was well received by nursing staff and physicians. Because nursing is a dynamic profession, practice has evolved so that today in some states RNs are permitted to pronounce patients.

It is critical that all RNs understand the rules, regulations and scope of practice in the state in which they're practicing including independent, dependent and interdependent practice. Your ability to frame your conversations with members of the interdisciplinary team will often depend on how well you understand and articulate these practice concepts. Your professional confidence and competence will guide the breadth and depth of your practice, as well as your ability to articulate your role as an RN.

Nursing Practice in Action

In the fall of 1995, ANA published the *Report Card on Nursing Practice*, identifying 35 indicators that were considered nurse-sensitive. Nurse-sensitive outcomes are elements of patient care directly affected by nursing practice. Nurse leaders in California embraced this work. By January 1996, leaders from more than 20 professional nursing organizations came together to identify which indicators should be adopted in acute care facilities across the state. From those early meetings, the California Nursing Outcomes Coalition was born.

Today, the registry has grown to 300 hospitals in nine states and is now known as the Collaborative Alliance for Nursing Outcomes (CALNOC). Nurse researchers, administrators and direct care registered nurses collect data on several nurse-sensitive indicators through CALNOC. This work has resulted in the improvement of patient care across the continuum, especially in the areas of hospital-acquired pressure ulcers and falls.

Many best practices are the result of nurses' independent practice. For example, the assessment tools developed to determine a patient's risk for falls or pressure ulcers are independent practice functions. The plan of care we implement as a result of the assessment may include independent, dependent and interdependent practice.

Independent practice for patients identified at risk for falls may include hourly rounding, implementing signage to indicate to the team that the patient is at risk and educating the family about preventing falls at home. Dependent functions may include the need for specific orders such as a physical therapy evaluation or medication adjustment. Interdependent practice would include implementation of a standardized procedure that your facility adopts to meet the care needs of this particular patient population.

Putting It All Together

As a professional nurse you'll continue to add to your toolkit throughout your career. Your practice will be influenced by current research, professional standards of practice and your personal commitment to improve the care you provide to your patients.

Nurses who are grounded in professional practice make every patient interaction a meaningful moment. Bath time is an opportunity to assess the patient's skin, mobility and functional status. Medication administration enables the nurse to assess the patient's hand-eye coordination, swallowing ability and cognitive status. Ambulation is an opportunity for interdisciplinary collaboration as we work with the physical therapist or pulmonary reconditioning team. Every patient interaction becomes a teaching moment for the patient and family, as well as students and other members of the interdisciplinary team.

Throughout this chapter, we've helped you understand your practice from a legal and professional perspective. Even with a keen understanding of your state's practice act, standards of performance, your employer's standards and your specialty in nursing, issues will inevitably surface that will cause you to pause.

These are the times you must listen to your inner voice, ask questions and evaluate the response. If your intuition tells you something doesn't seem right – take a time out. Ask your preceptor or a colleague to help you identify what's going on. You may not know the answer, but your intuition should not be ignored.

Never forget it is an honor and privilege to practice nursing. We enter people's lives at their most vulnerable times. Our compassion and competence will be instrumental in their journey, regardless of where it takes them.

Evolving as a Professional RN

Pat shares this story:

As a new graduate, I was frequently rewarded for the procedures/tasks I performed. I had the unique ability to run the Harvard Pump (a specialized machine generally used to administer medications directly into the hepatic artery) without the dreaded leakage. I could assemble the 10 sections of high pressure tubing needed for Swan Ganz catheters faster and more accurately than the senior nurses. The system I devised to ensure that I completed and recorded patient assessments gained the attention and support of my supervisors.

In retrospect, I realized that I was a great task-oriented nurse. It took some great mentors, an appreciation for the *California Nurse Practice Act*, the American Nurses Association's *Standards of Practice* and *Code of Ethics* as well as a commitment to lifelong learning before I could truly say I was practicing as a professional registered nurse.

While in nursing school, I learned the nursing process. I used it when assessing and planning care for my patients. However, I don't believe I fully appreciated the power of this tool in my early days as an RN. I know that I failed on more than one occasion to utilize the final step of the process – that of evaluating my interventions and patients' responses to those interventions. It took a few years in practice before I truly learned to appreciate that my critical thinking expertise was directly related to my use of the nursing process.

I was very fortunate in my early career to have an excellent mentor who challenged and encouraged me. Ellen was our associate director of nursing. She had been the chief nursing officer at a large hospital in California, an educator in Hawaii and served in a combined academic and service role in New Jersey. To me, she was the epitome of a truly seasoned professional nurse.

Each day with a red pencil behind her ear, Ellen would round on all the critical care patients. The red pencil was her way of documenting professional nursing practice ideas and strategies. I would provide her with a detailed report on my patients. Very quietly she would ask me questions about each patient's goals and their response to nursing interventions. While she asked these questions, I would be thinking: *Patient goals – my patients are intubated or comatose – wasn't she listening to me?*

This questioning would go on every day, until one day she just took notes. Her questions had forced me to look at my practice differently. I began to frame my report by beginning with the stability of the patient and concluding with their long-term goal. Ellen also helped me reframe my conversations with my peers and members of the health care team.

Just as I was grasping the importance of professional nursing practice, I started my BSN/MSN program. The program's faculty further challenged my thinking by teaching me that as RNs we have three dimensions to our role on the health care team. My mentors helped me see that, like all health care professional disciplines, we are first professionals, then registered nurses and finally we are members of the health care team serving the patient in a specific role or position. Our role on the health care team may change during our nursing careers, but we're always professionals and registered nurses. Under my mentors' guidance, I truly began to appreciate our state's *Nurse Practice Act* and the privileges of being an RN.

It is through formal and informal education, as well as our experiences and maturity, that bring depth to how we practice as professional registered nurses. As you progress on the novice to expert continuum, you'll develop a deeper understanding of your role as a professional nurse. I'm very proud to say that after nearly 40 years of practice, I remain as committed to nursing today as I was that first time I signed RN after my name.

Questions for Reflection

1. Review your state's nurse practice act. Does your state have a combined RN and LVN (LPN) practice act or separate regulations? What does your state practice act say about RN supervision of the LVN (LPN) and unlicensed assistive personnel?

Now review your job description, along with the job descriptions for LVNs (LPNs) and unlicensed assistive personnel. Do the job descriptions support the board's position on supervision?

2. How does your state practice act address independent practice? What are the required steps needed to develop a standardized procedure or procedure for overlapping or interdependent practice? Who can implement standardized procedures/policies related to overlapping or interdependent practice? What are the approved procedures or policies addressing overlapping practice for your facility's nursing department?

3. Consider your practice – is there an issue that you think could be addressed by developing a standardized procedure or policy on overlapping practice? How would you go about moving this idea forward for consideration?

4. Jan is working on the medical unit when her neighbor, Beth, is admitted to another unit in the same hospital. That evening, Jan is at her son's baseball game when some of the neighbors begin talking about Beth. They're concerned about Beth's condition and want to help. One of them asks Jan to check on how Beth is doing and keep them updated. If you were Jan, what would you do?

5. A famous sports figure has been admitted to your unit under an alias to protect his privacy. News of his admission has been reported on TV and *Facebook*. The outside world is buzzing about his condition. Staff from other departments are calling your unit to get the scoop. What do you do?

Communication Skills: The Foundation of Your Success as an RN

"If you just communicate you can get by. But if you skillfully communicate you can work miracles."

John Rohn

As a new graduate RN, you're focused on building your expertise in many areas – technical skills, diagnoses, critical thinking, leadership, and policies and procedures to name a few. However, one often overlooked skill that's a major factor in determining your success as a nurse, team member and new employee is your ability to communicate effectively.

Effective communication is a skill often taken for granted and not emphasized nearly as much as it should be. This skill is critical, not only for your success, but also for the safety of your patients.

Research clearly shows that the majority of medical errors are related to poor communication. Sometimes it's because instructions are ineffectively communicated and, as a result, are misinterpreted. At other times, assumptions are made to fill in gaps in communication and the assumptions prove to be incorrect. Or perhaps, people are afraid to stand up to a disruptive physician or team member, and don't speak up when they see something wrong. The result: errors that harm our patients. Because communication is such a huge factor in prevention of medical errors, several of The Joint Commission's *National Patient Safety Goals* contain effective communication with patients and/or among staff as part of their performance standards.

In addition, your verbal and nonverbal communication with your patients and their families can make a huge difference in how they cope with illness and treatments. Your relationship with your manager and fellow team members can determine your success and level of happiness as a new employee. These relationships can be greatly enhanced by good, consistent communication.

Just like any other skill – starting IVs, giving injections and assessing patients – your prowess as a communicator will grow with practice. In this chapter, we start with the building blocks of good communication. In the following chapter, we take these communication concepts and show you how to apply them to handle difficult conversations, resolve conflict, give effective feedback and deal with disruptive behavior.

Communication 101

To improve your communication skills, you must first have a fundamental understanding of how communication works at the basic level.

The *Communication Loop* below represents the foundation of all communication. When you have difficulty communicating with others, whether they're patients, family members or colleagues, always refer back to the fundamentals of the *Communication Loop*. Remembering these basic principles can help you get your interaction back on track.

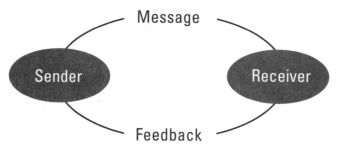

Here's how it works:

In any communication, there is a *message* (the information being conveyed), a *sender* (who initiates the message) and a *receiver* (who is the intended recipient). For the communication to be successful, the message must be received. The sender confirms that the message is received through *feedback*. This can be verbal acknowledgement of the message and/or nonverbal cues, such as nodding of the head, facial expressions, etc.

The key concept is that if the message is not received, then there is no communication. This is one of the main reasons many communications fail. Just because a sender conveys a message, this doesn't mean the message was received and/or understood. The most obvious example of this concept is speaking to someone in a foreign language that they don't understand. They don't have any idea what the message is, and as a result, this is a failed communication.

At this point, you may be thinking: *That's obvious! Tell me something I don't know to help me become a better communicator.*

Well, let's take this concept and see how it plays out in some common examples that occur daily in nursing and health care:

• Your patient is in pain, yet you begin to discuss his upcoming surgery because you need to get the consent form signed. *Is he really hearing and understanding or is his pain a barrier to your message?*

• A physician is talking to a patient about their condition, treatment and prognosis. The MD is using many technical terms, even though the patient has no health care background. *Does the patient really understand what was just said?*

• Your patient's wife is very worried and anxious about her husband's condition. You can see that her hands are shaking and she's on the verge of tears. You attempt to explain his condition and what his course of treatment will be. *Will the wife's distraught emotional state allow her to take in and comprehend this information?*

• One of your co-workers was just yelled at by a physician in front of other staff members. She is visibly angry and upset. You try to convey a message from the lab about a critical value for one of her patients. *Is she focused on what you're saying or on her own anger and embarrassment?*

• Your manager is walking rapidly through the unit. He says he's late for a meeting where he must give a presentation. You follow him to the elevator to ask permission to make a schedule change. *Is his mind on his meeting and presentation or your message?*

In how many of these examples do you think the message was received? If you said none, you're probably correct. When people are emotional, uncomfortable, in a hurry and/or deeply focused on what they feel is a pressing issue, they will most likely tune out any messages they think are less important than what they're currently experiencing. Or perhaps they'll remember a piece of the message – but is it the important piece or have they lost the meaning of what you were trying to say? So many times, people assume because they sent the message, it was effectively communicated. But that's only one step in the process. The communication isn't effective unless the message is fully received.

When conversing with others, focus on this key concept to hone your skills as a communicator. When you're the sender, make sure your message was received and understood by paying attention to verbal and nonverbal feedback by the other person. When you're the receiver of a message, ensure that you fully comprehend the message and meaning behind it.

"Of all the insights I've had into nursing during my first year, the greatest was my realization that the RN is a nerve center, the main link between the patient and everyone else." Chris Poole

Read Chris' story, *The Nerve Center*, on page 244.

Awareness of Self and Others

According to Sherod Miller, et al, author of *Connecting with Self and Others*, one of the first steps in becoming a more effective communicator is to develop a better understanding of yourself and the people you're communicating with. Miller explains:

"Your personal power increases with awareness. The more you can know about yourself and others at any moment, the more effective you will become in completing communications and bridging impasses in a wide variety of critical situations. You can be the person to make the difference. You can initiate change."

According to Miller, there are five key areas to consider when striving to better understand your personal communication style and the style of others:

Sensory Data – We connect with the world around us through our senses. The actions and messages of the people we communicate with are our sensory input. Build your awareness by paying closer attention to the sensory data you receive as you communicate. Also think about what sensory data you send out. Are you speaking clearly? Is the vocabulary you're using appropriate for the situation? What are your nonverbal messages? (More about nonverbal communication later in this chapter).

Thoughts – This is the meaning we make of the sensory data we take in. How we interpret and make meaning out of data depends on many factors, including our beliefs, values, expectations, personality and past experiences.

Feelings – These are our emotional responses to the situation. Being able to better connect with feelings – yours and others – is central to effective communication.

Wants – Our desires and intentions for ourselves and others. Our wants usually reflect our core values and include what we aspire to be and hope to accomplish. Our wants drive our actions.

Actions – This is our behavior, which is motivated by the previous four categories. This is the point where each of us makes choices about what to do or say (or not do or say).

Take a moment to think about this. When you or another person take action, it's based on: sensory data collected, how the information is interpreted, emotional responses to this interpretation and basic desires and intentions. Can you see how miscommunications can occur so easily? Two people can experience the same situation, yet react differently. Perhaps one person derives a different meaning from the sensory data than someone else. Maybe the situation evokes anger in one person and indifference in another. Or someone wants something totally different than the others involved.

There are many possibilities. But by increasing your awareness of your own style and what drives the actions of others, you can greatly enhance your ability to effectively communicate.

Let's explore this further by expanding on some of the factors that will help you better understand yourself and others.

Personality

Our individual personality provides a basic foundation for how we interpret and react to sensory data, and is an influential force in our resulting actions and communication.

Dictionary.com defines personality as the "visible aspects of one's character; the sum total of the physical, mental, emotional and social characteristics of an individual."

Observing and understanding human behavior and personality dates as far back as 460 BC when Hippocrates began describing and categorizing people's basic "humors" or approaches to life. Since that time, several psychologists and scientists have studied and described personality. Some of the most notable include: Carl Jung, David Keirsey, Katherine Myers and Isabel Briggs.

In continuing our discussion about personality and behavior, we will utilize the work of Don Lowry and his model – *True Colors*. Originally introduced in 1978, *True Colors* is widely used today as an easy, accurate and fun way to learn more about personality and behavior. The *True Colors* personality inventory is categorized by four colors: blue, gold, orange and green. Each color corresponds to a set of personality traits or characteristics.

Learning About Your Personality and Behavior Through *True Colors*

A Few Points to Remember Before We Talk About Personality

When we discuss and describe personality inventories, types and characteristics, this isn't an attempt to categorize people and fit them neatly into boxes. No one fits completely and exclusively into one category.

Although one personality type is usually the most dominant, we all have traits from different categories or colors and in differing levels of intensity. No one displays all the attributes of a color, even if it's their predominant one. Also, as we discuss throughout this chapter, who we are is dependent on a wide variety of factors with personality being only one of them.

When we talk about roles or professions related to color types, we mean that people with the personality traits of that particular color are often attracted to certain professions. For example, a high percentage of nurses have blue as a dominant color. This doesn't mean that in order to be a good nurse you must display traits predominately from the blue category. However, people with many of the blue personality traits are attracted to helping/service professions such as nursing.

Finally, no one personality type is right or wrong or better or worse than another. The goal of learning more about personality is to enhance understanding of ourselves and others. This will ultimately enable you to communicate more consistently and effectively and build positive relationships.

The following information about the *True Colors* system is based on the books: *Showing Your True Colors* by Mary Miscisin and *Living Your True Colors* by Tom Maddron, and information from the *True Colors* website (truecolorsintl.com).

BLUE: People-Oriented, Optimistic, Creative

Those with the predominate color of *Blue* highly value people and relationships. They're enthusiastic, optimistic and tend to "look on the bright side." *Blues* are often generous, nurturing and sensitive to the needs of others. They can be found in the helping professions, such as nursing, social work and teaching. Many *Blues* deplore injustice and unfairness, and passionately take up causes they believe will better the lives of others. Self expression is important to those *Blues* who are creative and aspire to be unique.

People with a predominately *Blue* personality can be sensitive and may display emotional outbursts and/or suffer from frequent hurt feelings. Because they value harmony, *Blues* will often avoid conflict and shy away from speaking the truth – afraid they might hurt someone's feelings. They often take on too much, sometimes reaching the point of overload, again because they don't want to hurt another person's feelings by saying no.

Blues often view themselves as: caring, flexible, passionate and friendly, with a strong desire to improve the lives of others.

Other colors may see *Blues* as: emotional, overly sensitive, indecisive and/or unrealistic.

For example: Barb has been an oncology nurse for 14 years. She is described by her patients and peers as extremely caring and compassionate. Whenever possible, she wears bright colors and is often smiling. Barb says this is good for patient morale. Although Barb has a professional demeanor, her manager and coworkers are concerned that she sometimes becomes "too emotionally involved" with her patients – they're worried this may result in compassion fatigue. When staffing is short, Barb is one of the first RNs called because her peers know she's ususally willing to help out, even if she would prefer not to work that day. Some staff members often ask Barb for help even if she's busy because they know she rarely says no. But when she becomes too overwhelmed, Barb has been known to act out in anger at others. Barb is very committed to the causes she believes in. She volunteers at a local soup kitchen, is active in her professional nursing organization and passionately engages in discussions about political and social issues.

GOLD: Consistent, Organized, Responsible

Always prepared, those who exhibit strong *Gold* traits tend to be extremely organized and detail oriented. They have a strong sense of duty and are conscientious, loyal and punctual. They value consistency and tradition. Some of the job roles that attract *Golds* are: pharmacists, accountants and attorneys.

Golds are often linear thinkers and therefore are proponents of rules, policies, checklists, etc. They can become impatient with people who break or bend rules or don't follow established procedures. They're most comfortable in a structured environment, and can be more resistant to change than other colors. *Golds* generally don't like doing things at the last minute, and may be uncomfortable working with people who are more spontaneous.

Golds often view themselves as: stable, dependable, efficient, responsible and punctual.

Other colors may see *Golds* as: rigid, uptight, uncompromising and/or judgmental.

For example: Sandy is a nurse on the respiratory telemetry unit. She loves patient care, especially organizing all of the nursing tasks and patient needs so the shift flows smoothly. Sandy created a grid that she uses to organize her patient assignments and tasks so she doesn't miss anything. She makes sure her patients' rooms are neat and tidy – for the safety of the patients and because she can't stand clutter. Sandy takes pride in wearing predominately white uniforms that are clean, neat and wrinkle free. She thinks that some of her RN colleagues dress too casually and don't look professional. Sandy enjoys collecting data and has been involved in several quality improvement projects in her department. However, she becomes frustrated because some of the other RNs often don't conform to the established policies and procedures. She's watching the job postings and is considering applying for a job in quality when one opens up. Outside of work, Sandy spends much of her time with family, and attending social functions and events at their church.

ORANGE: Action-Oriented, Spontaneous, Risk-Taker

Those exhibiting predominately *Orange* personality traits are often very energetic and action-oriented. Unlike *Golds* who value stability and consistency, *Oranges* thrive on change, challenge and spontaneity. The status quo is boring to them. Instead, *Oranges* like to push the envelope and take risks in order to keep moving forward and make improvements. *Oranges* can be quick-witted and charming, which makes them excellent communicators, negotiators and mediators. Many leaders in executive positions and entrepreneurs have strong *Orange* tendencies. The combination of their risk-taking, charm, adaptability and willingness to accept challenges can be great assets as they climb corporate ladders.

Because *Oranges* tend to be spontaneous and make quick decisions, they don't always consider all the relevant facts and pieces of the puzzle before taking action. Their attention span is limited. If the message they're receiving isn't short and to the point, they may quickly tune others out and not get all the facts.

Oranges often view themselves as: friendly, spontaneous, fun-loving, successful and good leaders.

Other colors may see *Oranges* as: impatient, irresponsible, manipulative, easily distracted and/or unprepared.

For example: George is an emergency department nurse. He loves the chaos and excitement of the ED, because you never know what type of patient will come through the door. He spent two years on the med/surg floor and became bored by the routine. He works part-time in the ED and part-time as a critical care transport RN for an ambulance company. He volunteers for extra projects and activities in the ED, as long as it doesn't involve serving on a committee. Committee meetings are often so tedious. George strives to be on time for work, but isn't very punctual in his personal life – much to the chagrin of his girlfriend. He doesn't understand why she reacts that way, and wishes she'd be more spontaneous. In his spare time, George likes to rock climb, snow board and surf. He is very excited because next weekend he's going sky diving for the first time.

GREEN: Competent, Analytical, Logical

People who express predominately *Green* traits are often very complex. Unlike *Blues*, who are comfortable with feelings and emotions, *Greens* find solace in problem-solving and intellectual pursuits. Generally, *Greens* view emotions as hindering the process of problem-solving. They like to expand their knowledge through research, analysis and asking questions. They're very comfortable working independently, and don't necessarily need the company of others. *Greens* are usually calm when others are anxious or emotional. *Greens* are often visionary and big picture thinkers. Careers that attract the *Green* personality include physicians, scientists and engineers.

Of the four colors, *Green* personalities are often the most misunderstood by others. Their lack of emotional expression is sometimes misinterpreted as being cold and insensitive. Their sense of humor tends to be on the sarcastic side, which at times may seem insulting to others. Because they like to thoroughly analyze a situation before making a decision, they may be slow to act in some circumstances. However, when they do make a decision, it's usually well thought out taking into account all possible options.

Greens often view themselves as: knowledgeable, rational, innovative, visionary and witty.

Other colors may see *Greens* as: arrogant, insensitive, eccentric, aloof and/or critical.

For example: Dr. Hughes is a neurologist. He enjoys the challenges and scientific aspects of being a physician, especially when he successfully diagnoses and treats a complex condition. Despite his success as a physician, he is sometimes uncomfortable interacting with his patients. He feels frustrated when they ask too many questions after he's already explained their condition and treatment. In the hospital, Dr. Hughes recognizes that nurses play an important role, but sometimes he is short-tempered when they call him with what he considers trivial questions. He doesn't like to attend social functions, and instead prefers spending his leisure time catching up on his journal articles, tinkering with his computer or working on his car. When his wife drags him to a party, he often finds a spot in the corner and observes others or plays games on his smart phone. He has a wry sense of humor. Most of his physician friends appreciate his humorous comments, so he's very surprised when others are offended by what he thinks are witty remarks.

The sample profiles described previously are intended to illustrate some of the major characteristics of the various colors. Barb, Sandy, George and Dr. Hughes are fictitious characters. If they were real people, in addition to their predominate personality style, they would also display characteristics and traits from the other colors as well. As we've said before, none of us has exclusively one personality style. We exhibit a variety of characteristics and traits.

In order to be successful, many of us have learned to cultivate some of the traits or qualities that don't come as naturally to us. Barb may learn to say "no" more often as a defense mechanism so she won't feel overwhelmed by taking on too many tasks. To decrease her frustration on the job, Sandy may try to accept that her colleagues don't practice nursing exactly the same way she does, but they still get the job done. George may try to be on time more often to avoid arguments with his girlfriend. Dr. Hughes may make more of an effort to connect with his patients when conversing with them in order to build a stronger doctor-patient relationship.

Building Stronger Relationships Through a Better Understanding of Personality

Recognizing your personality traits and those of others will help you build stronger relationships and enhance your communication skills. Seeing the similarities and differences helps you realize that, although you have many areas of commonality with others, you also may have different styles, outlooks and ways of accomplishing goals and tasks. So if someone reacts differently than you would in a particular situation, it's not because they don't like you or are trying to annoy you. It's usually because they see things differently than you.

Not wrong – just different!

Each of us is a unique individual. What makes us unique is our combination of personality traits and other factors we will discuss in the coming pages. By building awareness of the various aspects of your personality, you can maximize your strengths and identify areas you'd like to improve. Recognizing the personality traits of others will help you build a better understanding of those you interact with and ultimately enhance your effectiveness as a communicator.

Extrovert or Introvert?

Another factor to consider is whether an individual is extroverted or introverted. Just as we discussed regarding personalities, no one is exclusively introverted or extroverted, yet each of us has a predominate style. Your style may depend on the situation or setting. Some people are extroverted in social situations, but introverted in the work setting – or vice versa. Let's take a closer look at these two concepts.

Extroverts gain energy from external stimuli. They're very outgoing and like to interact with others. The more an extrovert is surrounded by other people, the more their energy increases and the happier they are. Extroverts enjoy social situations and will seek them out. They prefer to be with people rather than being alone. They often say exactly what's on their minds without thinking about it first, which can sometimes get them into trouble.

Conversely, introverts derive energy from within. They prefer to think and reflect prior to sharing their opinions. They're content spending time alone. Large groups of people make them feel uncomfortable – instead they prefer a small, close circle of friends. Although usually quiet in settings with new or large numbers of people, they can be very talkative with their close circle. Too much interaction with others can be draining to an introvert, and they need private time to re-energize.

Here's an example:

Sharon and Becky work the 12-hour day shift in the ICU. Today was a particularly hectic shift, and both of them, along with their colleagues are dragging a bit at the end of the day. Sharon says: "C'mon everybody, let's go to that new place down the street and get a drink. If we hurry, we can still get there before Happy Hour ends."

Becky replies: "I've heard that place is really crowded."

"That's why it's so fun," says Sharon. "You never know who you're going to meet!"

"You all go ahead," says Becky. "Jim has a meeting tonight, and I'm looking forward to spending some time alone with the new mystery novel I just bought."

"That sounds really boring," Sharon mumbles as she and two others hurry out the door to get to Happy Hour.

This is an obvious example, but you get the idea. Sharon, the extrovert, is energized by going with her friends to a crowded place where she also has the prospect of meeting new people. On the other hand, introverted Becky is looking forward to some quiet time in order to recharge her batteries.

How does extroversion versus introversion affect personality and communication? The personality traits we discussed in *True Colors* will usually be more easily recognizable in an extroverted person, whereas, they might not be so easy to spot in an introvert.

Generational Differences

As you build awareness of yourself and others, another important factor to consider is the generational differences between you and the person you're communicating with. Most sources describe four generational categories in today's workforce. Although there are similarities between all groups, there are also some major differences in values, motivations, beliefs, influences and driving forces. A general understanding of the differences between generations can enhance your ability to communicate with a wide variety of people. Let's take a brief look at some of the key descriptors of each generation.

Depending on the sources utilized, the birth years depicting a particular generation can vary. For the purposes of our discussion, we are basing the information presented below predominately from the research of Ron Zemke et al., as described in the book *Generations at Work*.

Traditionals/Veterans/Matures, *born between 1922 and 1943*

Most of the members of this generation are retired. Greatly influenced by the Great Depression and World War II, *Traditionals* are generally conservative, adverse to risk and highly disciplined with a strong sense of obligation. In the workplace, they respect authority, prefer hierarchical leadership and adhere to the chain of command. Consistent, loyal and patient, they believe in "paying your dues" in order to get ahead. Many spent most or all of their careers working for one company. They value teamwork and collaboration and are often uncomfortable with conflict.

Because of their strong respect for authority, patients of the *Traditional* generation are uncomfortable advocating for their health care needs and often will not question decisions or advice of their physicians and other members of the health care team. In addition, they may not readily complain of pain or discomfort, unwilling to be a bother to others.

Baby Boomers, *born between 1943 and 1960*

This generation has the largest number of members. Therefore, they have a great impact on business, politics and consumer goods. Many *Boomers* were significantly influenced by the tumultuous events of the 1960s, including the Vietnam War, the civil rights movement, landing on the moon, the sexual revolution and the assassinations of key public figures including John and Robert Kennedy and Martin Luther King. Although raised to respect authority by their traditionalist parents, many *Boomers*, as college students and young adults, publicly protested government decisions and those in authority.

In the workplace, many leadership positions are held by *Boomers*. They are goal-oriented, competitive and believe in hard work and sacrifice. The phrase "workaholic" was coined to describe their long work hours and determination to succeed. *Boomers* are confident, optimistic and value job security. They tend to be materialistic and some have a strong sense of entitlement. They value health, personal growth and gratification. *Boomers* also value relationships and prefer to avoid conflict whenever possible. When communicating, they like some constructive feedback, but are put off by frequent appraisal.

In the health care setting, it's important to note that *Baby Boomers* are sometimes also called the "sandwich generation" because many are attempting to care for aging parents as well as their own children. This can be highly stressful for these *Boomers,* and may impact their health.

Generation Xers, *born between 1960 and 1980*

These are the children of older *Boomers*. *GenXers* grew up honing their survival instincts and skills as many of them were "latchkey" kids, coming home from school with no adult supervision in the house. This was usually because both parents were working or they lived in a single parent household. Older kids cared for their younger siblings. There were several negative historical events during their formative years, including: the loss of the Vietnam War; Watergate and the resulting resignation of President Nixon, who was later pardoned by his appointed successor; and the outbreak of AIDS. They were also greatly influenced by MTV and global competition.

In the workplace, *GenXers* are independent, confident and self-reliant. Although they want to earn a good salary, many *Xers* more highly value work-life balance, flexible work schedules and stimulating, pleasant work. Unlike the *Traditionals* and *Boomers*, *Xers* generally don't have a high level of loyalty to their employers, but are extremely loyal to family and friends. They are results-oriented, believing that accomplishments should outweigh time spent at work. They value lifelong learning and skill development. *GenXers* aren't intimidated by authority and will speak out with suggestions, questions or problems. They prefer both giving and receiving immediate and continuous feedback.

In the health care setting, they will ask many questions, play an active role in their treatment and learn as much as they can about medical conditions affecting themselves and their loved ones.

Millenials, Generation Y, *born between 1980 and 2000*

The newest generation in the workforce, *Millenials* share some of the values and characteristics of *GenXers*. They've been greatly influenced by rapid technological advances – computers, video games, iPods and smart phones. They're very comfortable with these high-tech devices and are excellent multi-taskers, especially utilizing multiple technologies simultaneously. They communicate freely using online tools, however, they can sometimes be unskilled and uncomfortable with face-to-face communication.

Millenials are the most highly educated generation, recognizing the value of learning to further their goals. They are optimistic and adaptable to change. In the workplace, *Millenials* value teamwork, collective action and diversity. Loyalty to their employer is often based on their commitment to the company's mission, values and products or services. Many seek organizations aligned with their own values.

Some characterize *Millenials* as demanding, but they're confident and know what they want. They prefer immediate and frequent feedback. In the health care setting, *Millenials* strive to play an active role in their health and wellness.

Awareness of Culture

In addition to personality and generational considerations, another key component in your quest to better understand yourself and others is increased awareness of the beliefs and practices of people from diverse cultures – and how this can affect behavior and influence communication.

Most health care settings are filled with both patients and staff representing diverse cultures. As a nurse, you've probably been exposed to information and training to help build your "cultural competence" as a patient care provider. This is important education and an initial step in shaping your understanding of people with varying ethnic origins. However, often overlooked is building an understanding and strategy for effectively communicating with your co-workers from differing cultures.

Failing to understand and appreciate the beliefs, values, perspectives and communication styles of people from diverse backgrounds can result in miscommunication and conflict. Outlined below are some general examples of communication styles among varying cultures. Once again, this is not an attempt to categorize or stereotype people. The goal is to build awareness of differing styles in order to enhance communication.

- Coworkers from other countries may speak English, but can still have difficulty understanding the nuances, such as implied meaning, slang, context and generational and regional variations of the English being spoken in the workplace.

- Different cultures have varying views regarding eye contact and personal space. Some maintain eye contact and stand close to the person they're talking to. For other cultures, prolonged eye contact is considered disrespectful. Standing too close may be regarded as an invasion of personal space and, as a result, can be uncomfortable and hinder communication.

- Some Asian cultures value harmony, and therefore will often remain silent in difficult situations, rather than risk a conflict.

- In the US workplace, punctuality and productivity are highly valued. Other cultures may not be as time-centric and consider maintaining personal relationships more valuable than punctuality.

These are just a few basic examples of differences among diverse cultures. As you strive to learn more about people from other cultures, Juliene Lipson and Suzanne Dibble, authors of *Culture and Clinical Care*, caution against stereotyping – applying cultural facts indiscriminately to everyone from a particular ethnic group, rather than learning whether or not an individual fits those suppositions. Instead, Lipson and Dibble recommend generalizing – beginning with a supposition about a group as a first step, then striving to learn whether these characteristics indeed fit an individual from that group. Learning generalized information about a particular ethnic group is only the beginning of understanding.

"I want to care for and support families as they experience the most scary and challenging times in their lives." Sara Glass

Read Sara's story, *Breaking Through the "Difficult" Facade*, on page 188.

Learning More about Your Patients from Diverse Cultures

• Take time to learn about other cultures. Begin with the most prevalent cultures in your health care organization's patient population. Read about these cultures; respectfully ask patients questions about their beliefs, customs and practices.

• Don't appear judgmental if the patients and/or their family members want to utilize nontraditional medical practices as part of the treatment. For example, in some cultures certain foods are given to loved ones suffering from fever. These foods are believed to bring the body's temperature back to normal. Allowing these practices can enhance your patient's comfort and their healing environment.

• Use certified medical interpreters when communicating with patients who speak little or no English to discuss diagnosis, treatment options, medications, procedures, discharge instructions, etc. Although family members may be available, you won't know if they're filtering information to their loved ones. Additionally, patients may not share critical information about sensitive issues with family members. And as a health care provider, sharing certain information with the patient's family or friends may be a breach of confidentiality.

• In times of stress, people will return to their comfort zones. For English as a second language speakers, this comfort zone can be their native tongue – even if they speak English fluently. Ensure they're getting the information they need. You may need to call in an interpreter for assistance.

• If there is a language barrier, make sure the patient and family not only receive, but also comprehend, needed information. Don't assume that your patient understands information and instructions because they nod their head to signify yes. Some cultures will nod as a sign of politeness. They may also view asking questions as disrespectful or impolite, and might not ask even if they don't understand. If you're not sure the message was received, ask them questions to validate their understanding or utilize interpreter services.

Ensure Your Patients Receive and Understand the Message

Brenda shares this story:

My patient was a 60 year-old Latino male recovering from a myocardial infarction and subsequent coronary artery bypass surgery. He spoke little English and his wife spoke a moderate amount.

I entered his room one evening, and he and his wife were watching the health channel. The subject of the program was about adopting a heart healthy diet. As the program described in English what foods *NOT* to eat – thick steaks marbled with fat, butter, ice cream and cheeses with dark veins were pictured on the screen. My patient had a smile on his face. When I asked his wife why he was so happy, she replied that he was worried about sticking to a diet, "but he can live with this one!"

I immediately located the Spanish version of this educational program and played it for him. He wasn't so happy when he understood the actual parameters of his new diet. With the aid of an interpreter, I reinforced the message to make sure it was indeed received.

Bottom line: Ensure that your patients whose native language isn't English are getting the information and education they need to manage their conditions and improve their health.

Gaining a Better Understanding of Colleagues from Diverse Cultures

• As mentioned previously, learn more about the values, customs and beliefs of your colleagues. Ask questions about their cultural practices. Are there special holidays they celebrate? Describe and share your family's traditions and customs. A great place to start is with food. Some multi-cultural units have periodic potlucks where participants are encouraged to bring foods representing their cultures.

• Recognize and respect individual differences. Recognizing and respecting your colleagues from other cultures is a major step in enhancing communication.

• While accepting differences is important, so is looking for similarities. Although there are differences, you'll find that you have many things in common with your colleagues from diverse backgrounds.

• When communicating, look for nonverbal cues while listening to the words spoken. Does the person seem uncomfortable with sustained eye contact? Do they use certain gestures or facial expressions to convey anger, frustration, confusion, etc? As you pay more attention to a person's body language, you'll have better insight into the messages they're trying to convey. More about nonverbal communication later in this chapter.

• Recognize that English is a second language for some of your coworkers. Help them build their language skills by explaining slang expressions, speaking slowly and distinctly if they are having difficulty with a concept and being patient with them as they communicate.

"I learned that by making my own decision to be open-minded and positive, my shift turnd out to be a great learning experience." Kelly Navarro

Read Kelly's story, *Nothing is as Bad as it Seems,*, on page 228.

Make sure you and your coworkers have a common language for key words. For example, a travelling RN from Australia rushed out of a patient's room shouting: "I need the trolley! Someone get the trolley!" Her patient was on the verge of coding, and she wanted the crash cart in the patient's room. Because the other staff didn't associate the word "trolley" with the crash cart, they didn't respond until she explained what was happening. This wasted valuable time that would have been better spent aiding the emergent patient.

In this chapter, one of our goals is to increase your awareness of the many dynamics affecting communication. And culture is a huge factor. However, this was merely a brief overview of some major cultural considerations. In order to learn more, consult some of the many resources available to help build understanding and bridge communication among people of different cultures. And remember, the best way to learn more about someone is to ask them.

Nonverbal Communication

"What you do speaks so loud that I cannot hear what you say."
Ralph Waldo Emerson

We can't talk about the foundations of effective communication without including a discussion about nonverbal messages.

There are three components of a message: the words used, tone of voice and nonverbal messages. In the 1960s, communications researcher Dr. Albert Mehrabian conducted studies related to face-to-face communication and determined that these three components of communication had the following impact:

- 7% of the message received is from the spoken words.
- 38% of the message is received via the tone of voice, emphasis on certain words, whether speech is fast or slow, loud or soft, etc.
- 55% of the message is conveyed by nonverbals, such as facial expressions, mannerisms and body language.

While these statistics are quoted frequently, Dr. Mehrabian points out that his research is related to face-to-face conversations where feelings and attitudes are important. Furthermore, if a person's tone of voice and/or body language are incongruent with the words spoken, he found that the receiver of the message is much more likely to believe the nonverbal message, rather than the spoken words.

For example:

• You and Fred are expressing differing opinions about an issue. The discussion becomes heated, and you ask Fred if he's angry with you because you disagree with him. His response is: "NO, I am NOT mad at you!" His tone of voice and emphasis on the words "no" and "not" may tell you otherwise. What if in addition to his tone of voice, his face is red and he's pointing a finger at you. Now you're sure of it! Despite his words, Fred is angry.

• Kathy is your manager. You enter her office to ask if the department will fund your attendance at a conference out of state. You're well prepared and ready to describe the uses for the information you'll learn and bring back to share with fellow team members. You ask Kathy if she has a few minutes to talk. She says yes, but keeps glancing at her computer screen and her watch. Is this really a good time to discuss your important request with Kathy?

As you can see by these examples, paying attention to the way messages are delivered, as well as the body language and nonverbal cues that accompany the message, can be important signals to help you communicate more effectively.

What to Watch and Listen for:

Examples of Voice Cues

Tone of voice – Loud could signify anger or the intention to persuade or intimidate. A soft voice may convey sadness or uncertainty.

Pace – Fast may signify nervousness or emotion; stammering often signals confusion or possibly that the speaker is withholding key information.

Emphasis on certain words – As described in the example above regarding the heated discussion with Fred, emphasis on certain words can provide clues about true meaning and the other person's level of emotion.

Examples of Body Language

Posture – Is the person exhibiting a closed stance with arms folded, or is their stance open?

Facial expressions – Are they smiling or frowning? Making eye contact or avoiding it? Are their lips pursed? Does their lower lip seem relaxed, or is it tense or quivering? Are their face or cheeks becoming red or pale?

Gestures – Do their hand and arm gestures appear relaxed and are being used to emphasize a point? Or do the gestures convey agitation, excitement, frustration or anger?

The best way to improve your skills at interpreting nonverbals is to pay attention and practice. Look for groups of nonverbal signals that reinforce a general message. Be careful not to interpret nonverbal messages from only a single gesture. This often won't provide an accurate clue to the person's feelings and emotions. Also, nonverbals can be expressed differently depending on the individual. One person's facial expressions when they're concentrating may be misinterpreted by someone else as frowning, indicating anger or displeasure.

Let's look at an example:

Your manager stops you in the hallway to ask your opinion about an idea she has. The hallway is drafty, and as she begins to speak, you instinctively fold your arms against your chest in response to the chilly air. She becomes frustrated, saying that you are dismissing her idea without hearing her out. You're confused and initially have no idea why she's reacting this way. You think her idea is a good one. Finally, it comes out that your folded arms made her think you don't like her idea. You explain that your arms are folded because you're cold, not closed to her idea. It takes some persuasion to convince the manager that her interpretation of your body language doesn't accurately reflect your opinion.

If you think that someone's nonverbals don't match their message, seek clarification by asking. Let's revisit our previous examples with Fred and Kathy. Here are some possible responses to their nonverbal messages:

- "Fred, even though you say you're not, you appear angry to me. Are you? Is it what we're talking about, or is there something else going on?"

- "Kathy, you seem busy. Can I set a time to talk with you later this week? Would tomorrow at 3:30 when my shift ends work for you?"

Be aware of your own body language and the ways you deliver messages. Do your nonverbal cues support or disagree with your verbal messages? If you're not sure, practice an upcoming difficult conversation or presentation in front of the mirror. Pay attention to your facial expressions and gestures. Do they support your words or contradict them? Utilize gestures and expressions that clarify and support your words, so your meaning is conveyed accurately.

Legendary comedienne Lucille Ball spent hours each week practicing her *I Love Lucy* lines and jokes in front of large mirrors that showed every angle of her face and much of her body. She was continually searching for the facial expressions and gestures that would best complement her zany comedy routines and elicit the most laughs from her audiences. That practice and awareness of her nonverbal messages made her a huge success.

By paying attention to nonverbal messages and practicing your own skills, you too can significantly improve your ability to communicate effectively.

Listening

"I've learned to listen not just with my ears, but with my eyes and heart as well. Looking beyond the words people say allows me to respond to intuitive cues, which often more accurately reflect the speaker's message." Sandra Marken, BSN, RN

Think about the communication loop described at the beginning of this chapter. For communication to be effective, messages must not only be sent, but received. This is a two-way process, and a key element is listening. Just as we expect the other person to listen to us when we're talking, we must also listen to the other person in order to fully under-stand their message. Good listening also builds trust and strengthens your rapport with others.

Yet as important as good listening is, most listeners retain only 25-50 percent of what they hear.

"Mrs. G taught me to be an effective team leader by balancing clear and direct communication with strong listening skills." Kathy Harren

Read Kathy's story, *Better Care Through Effective Teams*, on page 250.

Building Your Listening Skills

Pay attention. Give the speaker your full attention. Make eye contact. Listen to the words spoken, but also take note of nonverbal messages.

Acknowledge the message. Use body language to show that you're listening, such as nodding, gesturing, using appropriate facial expressions. Also use verbal messages like *yes, I see, uh-huh*.

Periodically clarify information to confirm your understanding. Clarify information with phrases such as: "so what you're saying is…" Or, if you're unclear about the meaning, then ask a question: "What do you mean when you say…"

Don't interrupt with your point of view. Allow the speaker to finish before you give your opinion. If the communication is causing an emotional response in you, ask a clarifying question. In many cases, you may be misunderstanding what the speaker intended.

Respond appropriately and respectfully. Be honest and open when responding. Strive to remain calm and respectful, even if the other person becomes emotional or antagonistic. By role modeling a calm, respectful demeanor, hopefully the other person will de-escalate. Even if they don't, you'll be glad you were the one who stayed cool, calm and collected.

Keep practicing to build your skills. Listening sounds easy, but in reality it takes practice and determination, especially in difficult conversations or conflicts. Remind yourself to use these listening skills and soon they will become second nature.

Good Communication Takes Practice!

Although some are more skilled at communicating effectively than others, no one ever reaches perfection in this area. There is room for improvement for all of us. Keep practicing to build your skill at conveying effective messages, reading nonverbal cues, listening, and increasing your awareness of yourself and others. In the next chapter, we will apply this information to show you how to handle difficult conversations and resolve conflict.

As you move through your career, you'll find that building your communication skills is one of the single most effective strategies to help you attain personal and professional success.

Questions for Reflection

1. What are some strategies you can utilize to develop a better understanding of your communication style?

2. What are some ways you can strengthen you listening skills?

3. What specific steps can you take to become a better communicator?

4. You work with several RNs from the Baby Boomer generation. What are some of the characteristics of this generation? What can you do to communicate more effectively with this group?

5. What are the predominate cultures that make up the patient population in your facility? What can you do to learn more about the people from these cultures?

6. Review your organization's policy for interpreter services. When is it appropriate to utilize an interpreter? How do you access interpreter services in your health care organization?

Effective Communication Strategies for Challenging Situations

"Don't find fault. Find a remedy." Henry Ford

In the previous chapter, we described the major foundational elements of good communication. We discussed the importance of knowing yourself and understanding others; how personality, generation and culture influence behavior and communication; the impact of nonverbal messages; and the importance of listening. Now we're going to take these key concepts, add some other considerations, and apply this information to help you communicate effectively in difficult situations, resolve conflict positively, give appropriate and meaningful feedback to others and deal with disruptive behavior and bullying.

The following pages contain many concepts and tactics for addressing difficult communication situations. It may be too much to digest in one reading. Instead, we recommend reading a few concepts at a time and then pausing to reflect on the information. You may also need to read this chapter more than once to thoroughly grasp this information and develop a meaningful plan for its use. Our goal is to provide you with practical strategies you can employ to improve your communication skills in difficult situations.

Disruptive Behavior in the Health Care Workplace

Disruptive behavior (also called incivility, lateral violence or horizontal violence) is found to some degree in most workplaces, but can be especially prevalent in health care settings. The Joint Commission (JC), in *Sentinel Event Alert No. 40*, issued July 2008, stated that intimidating and disruptive behavior greatly contributes to medical errors and preventable adverse patient outcomes, increases the cost of care and causes some nurses to seek new employment or even leave the profession.

According to the JC, intimidating and disruptive behaviors consist of overt actions such as verbal outbursts and physical threats, as well as passive activities that include refusing to perform assigned tasks and exhibiting uncooperative behavior (see box below for more examples of disruptive behaviors).

Overt Disruptive Behavior
• Verbal outbursts
• Physical contact or threats
• Sabotage
• Intimidating comments

Passive/Subtle Disruptive Behavior
• Uncooperative attitudes
• Failure to return messages and pages
• Impatience with questions
• Condescending language or intonation
• Raising eyebrows, rolling eyes or other negative nonverbal messages
• Being disrespectful by belittling someone or using sarcastic put-downs
• Spreading rumors about others
• Excluding someone by deliberately conversing in a different language

The Joint Commission's issuance of a *Sentinel Event Alert* about disruptive behavior demonstrates the agency's belief in the severity of this problem and its negative impact on patient safety and workplace morale. Disruptive behavior can be especially intimidating to new graduate nurses, who already feel hesitant and unsure of themselves as they strive to learn and grow in their practice.

Some disruptive outbursts are reactions to acutely stressful situations, while other behavior may reflect deep-seated values, perceptions and biases. An individual responding negatively in a stressful situation, such as an emergency, may display disruptive behavior occasionally. They are often remorseful for their behavior, especially if it's brought to their attention. Whereas, a chronic intimidator will display disruptive behavior much more frequently, and often for no apparent reason.

Some individuals are unaware that their behavior is disruptive, especially when they see similar actions displayed by others in the workplace. Over time, they may have concluded that their aggressive style is an acceptable communication method in the health care environment. They are often shocked to learn that their conduct is a problem and has a negative impact on their patients and coworkers. Other individuals, commonly referred to as bullies, have no remorse for their actions or behavior and are purposefully intimidating and disruptive (we'll discuss bullying later in this chapter).

Dealing with Difficult Situations and People

Dealing with disruptive behavior sounds daunting! Even the Joint Commission recognizes this as a major problem affecting patient safety and employee satisfaction. You may be asking yourself: *What can I possibly do as one person to protect my patients and create a positive work environment?*

The answer is: *You can make a difference!* By resolving to address these situations as they occur and using positive communication strategies, you can create a more pleasant work environment and a stronger safety net for your patients. Let's look at several strategies to help you be successful.

Knowing Yourself and Others

Crucial Conversations, by Kerry Patterson, et al., provides strategies for resolving conflict and dealing with disruptive behavior which are widely used in health care and business settings. In *Crucial Conversations*, Patterson explains that when faced with an unresolved conflict or failed conversation, most of us are quick to blame others. *Look what they did...it's their fault.*

However in most cases, one party isn't totally guilty, and the other innocent. Both sides usually do something to contribute to the problem. Therefore, Patterson asserts, each person must start with their side of the equation – their role in the conflict. Ultimately, you can't change others, but you can change yourself and the way you respond when communicating in difficult situations.

In the last chapter we discussed ways to develop a better understanding of self and others. If we first understand ourselves – what motivates us, how we take in information and interpret it, what our communication style is and what we ultimately want from our interactions, we can refocus our efforts to realize our goals. Many effective communicators regularly examine and evaluate their responses in different circumstances to expand their self-awareness and improve their communication skills.

In addition to knowing yourself, if you work to increase your understanding of others, you can better comprehend, tolerate and respect individual differences. More importantly, you'll grow to recognize similarities – which you may find outnumber the differences. Before continuing with this chapter, you may want to revisit the previous chapter and review the material about building a better understanding of yourself and others.

Setting the Stage for Your Conversation

If you're planning to have an important conversation with someone or anticipate that the discussion may become sensitive or difficult, here are some steps to help you through the process:

• Review the situation or behavior you'd like to discuss ahead of time. Practice how you'll start the conversation.

• Determine what you want from the interaction and stay focused on those goals. If you have some anger or hurt feelings from a previous interaction with this person, look beyond those feelings and concentrate on achieving your desired outcomes.

• Consider how you think the other person will react. Prepare yourself for the most negative responses and your reactions to them. In most cases, the response is rarely as negative as we think it will be. But occasionally, the response will be just what you anticipated, or even more difficult. Hopefully, you'll find that as you practice these skills, your ability to predict the reactions of others and respond appropriately will improve.

• Approach the person in a calm and nonthreatening manner. Tell them you'd like to discuss something with them. Set up a mutually agreeable time for the discussion. Perhaps it's right now, or maybe it's later in your shift. If they're reluctant to set a time or vague about when they can meet ("we'll talk later"), set some parameters: *Sure, as long as we talk before we go home today.* Or: *We're both working tomorrow. Can we meet before our shift?*

• Meet in a private place, so that other team members can't hear the conversation. If someone else initiates a sensitive conversation with you in the presence of others, persuade them to move to a more private location.

Starting the Conversation

You have the person's attention. Now what? Your best bet is to stay focused on the issue at hand. This will help you avoid an angry or emotional outburst, and provides the best chance of resolving the issue. Always keep in mind your overall goal for having this conversation and what you'd like to accomplish.

Stay focused on the behavior or actions you observed and how these actions affect you. Don't make the conversation an attack on the individual.

Sherod Miller, in *Connecting with Self and Others*, suggests you start the dialogue like this:

When you: *(tell what happened, and what you observed)*

This resulted in: *(tell how the actions affected you or made you feel...)*

Next time: *(explain the action you'd like to see – your goal)*

Let's look at an example:

You're a new grad RN on the med/surg unit. You need to do a complicated dressing change on one of your post-op patients. You ask Marianne, one of the RNs on the unit, to assist you with the dressing change. Marianne agrees, tells you to gather the supplies and she'll meet you in the patient's room. You wait for 10 minutes and Marianne never comes. You look for Marianne, but can't find her, so you ask another nurse to assist you. This is the second time in a week that Marianne has agreed to help you and then not followed through. You decide you're going to talk to her about it.

You have a choice – make the issue a personal attack or try to address the problem in a nonthreatening way.

If you make the issue a personal attack:

"Marianne, what's your problem? I'd like to know what you've got against new grads? Or is it just me personally? This morning when I asked you to help me with Mr. Smith's dressing change, you told me to get the supplies and you'd meet me in his room. I waited for over 10 minutes and you never came. I looked like an idiot in front of my patient. But I guess that's what you wanted. I've heard from other people that you're out to get new grads..."

Obviously, this response illustrates the anger and frustration you're feeling (and probably some hurt feelings, too!). But approaching the conversation in this manner isn't going to solve the conflict. It leaves Marianne nowhere to go except to fight back or walk away. Certainly after being approached in this way, she's not going to apologize or see how her behavior disrupts your ability to care for your patients. So if you're still angry or emotional, don't have the conversation at that time. Wait until you cool off and can discuss the issue in a rational manner.

Now, let's approach the same situation in a nonthreatening way:

"Marianne, yesterday when I asked you to help me with Mr. Smith's dressing change, you told me to get the supplies and you'd meet me in his room. I waited for over 10 minutes and you never came. I had to scramble to find someone else to help me. The same thing happened last week when I asked you for help with another patient. Since this has happened twice in a week, I feel frustrated and this adds to my stress level. Next time, if you don't have time to help me, will you please tell me that when I ask?"

Now, wait for her response...

See the difference. You focused on the situation and how it made you feel rather than accusing Marianne of being out to get you and other new grads. You also described the behavior you'd like to see from now on when you ask Marianne for help.

Hopefully Marianne will say something like this:

"I'm sorry. I didn't mean to leave you waiting. Another patient needed something, and I got busy and forgot I was supposed to help you."

At this point, ideally, you can make a mutual agreement by saying: "Next time if you're busy, then perhaps I can help you and then you can help me." Marianne agrees to this.

It looks like the problem is resolved. But what if it happens again next week? It's tempting to throw your hands in the air and say behind her back: "I'm done trying to get along with her. Someday she's going to ask me for help, and there's no way I'm helping her." Or, you may decide to attack her personally.

Instead, stay focused on achieving what you want: to be able to count on Marianne as a fellow team member when you need help. So go right back to her, and calmly remind her of your agreement. Ask her why she once again said she'd help you and then didn't show up.

If Marianne knows you're going to hold her accountable for her agreement with you, she'll be less likely to break it. However, if you don't follow-up, she may think that you're hesitant to call her on her behavior. By not saying anything, you're sending the message to Marianne that her behavior is acceptable to you.

Pay Attention to What's Happening During the Conversation

How do you react in different situations? This again goes back to the importance of knowing yourself. What do you feel when a conversation becomes difficult – fast heart rate, butterflies in your stomach, dry mouth, shaky voice? Do you feel your lip quivering and that you may cry? In *Crucial Conversations*, Patterson says these are signals indicating to us a conversation is becoming difficult. These cues may also be a warning that we're about to move from a productive dialogue to an emotional response and a resulting negative outcome. Once you recognize these signals in yourself, you can use them to help you refocus and avoid an argument.

What messages are you sending to others? Do you become defensive if someone doesn't agree with you? Do you become angry? Are there specific triggers that set off your emotions? When you're in a conflict situation, what does your body language convey?

Notice how others are reacting in the conversation. Do they seem upset, angry, confused? If you're not getting the response you want, don't keep plowing forward. Read the cues and respond appropriately by asking questions, clarifying and/or changing the way you're delivering the message.

For example:

You are having a difficult conversation with Herman, today's charge nurse, about your patient assignment. When you arrived for your shift, you noticed that you've been assigned all new patients even though several of the patients you cared for yesterday are still on the unit. Herman and most of the other RNs haven't worked for the past few days. When you begin to tell him why you believe your assignment should be changed, Herman crosses his arms, rolls his eyes and sighs. By paying attention to these cues, you realize that you're not effectively getting your point across. This gives you the opportunity to use a different approach in explaining the need for your request. You can focus on continuity of care and the trust you built with your patients the day before. Or, you can ask a clarifying question about his response:

"I sense that you don't feel my request is valid. I'm here early, and the shift hasn't begun yet. I believe this assignment change will be better for the patients. Is there a reason why you don't think it's appropriate to adjust the assignment?"

Keep Your Emotions in Check

As stated earlier in this chapter, when faced with a failed conversation, many people are often quick to blame others. But in most cases, one party isn't totally at fault, and the other innocent. Both parties contribute to the problem – although some may have a bigger share than others. As we've stated over and over, to be effective communicators, each of us must first focus on ourselves and our responses.

Think about what you want from the conversation. If the person isn't responding the way you hoped they would, what are you going to do? If their response is negative, it can trigger an emotional response in you which negatively escalates the interaction. This could be lashing out verbally or using negative body language. These emotional responses will often derail the conversation, resulting in failure to accomplish desired outcomes and a strained relationship with the other person.

Strategies to Minimize Your Emotional Response

• Pause and take a deep breath. By pausing, even for a few seconds before responding, the urge to deliver an angry or emotional comeback often passes.

• Seek clarity so you know what the other person really meant by their statement. Did they really say something negative or hurtful, or is this your interpretation of their message? You can ask the question: What do you mean by that? Or, I don't understand why you said that to me, please explain. In some cases, the other person will realize that their response was inappropriate and will tone it down the second time around. After all, they're human too. They may have responded emotionally, and now wish they hadn't. How many times have you wished you could take back something you said? Or perhaps you misread their meaning and when they explain, you'll realize it wasn't an attack.

• Stay focused on your goals. If you respond emotionally, it may feel good for a short time, but is that response really going to get you what you want? The point is: you don't have to be the winner and the other person the loser to accomplish your goal. The best results usually occur in win-win situations.

• Whenever possible, keep the needs of the patient and/or the patient's family at the forefront. It's hard to argue against what's best for a patient. Staying focused on the patient can also help all parties keep their emotions in check.

• If you suspect ahead of time that the conversation is going to be difficult, set mutually agreed upon ground rules with the other person before discussing the issues. This will be an indication of your sincerity to make the conversation productive and reach a solution.

Let's look at an example:

You're a new graduate working in a high acuity unit and have been off orientation about two weeks. Although your confidence is growing, you're still nervous about caring for the patients with the highest acuity. As you're receiving report from Margot, the off-going nurse, you're feeling apprehensive because one of your patients has a diagnosis you're not very familiar with. You want to gain as much information as possible from Margot, so you ask her several questions about the patient's care.

Margot's responses are becoming short and curt. Suddenly, she snaps at you saying: "You new nurses – don't you know anything about caring for patients? I don't have time to train you now!"

Some of the people around you have stopped report and are looking at you. You are mortified...angry...embarrassed! Your first urge is to say something equally retaliatory. Something that will hurt her feelings, just as your feelings are hurt.

But what if you resist this urge? What if you pause, take a deep breath and remember what you want and why you asked the questions – to deliver safe care to a patient with a diagnosis you want to learn more about. Another of your goals is to be accepted as a valued member of the care team on your new unit.

Instead of the retaliatory response that your emotional side wants to fire at Margot, you pause to gain control of your emotions and calmly say: "I don't understand why you said that to me. Mr. Jones has a diagnosis we don't typically see on our unit, and I want to give him the best care I possibly can. Since you've been taking care of him all shift, I want to learn all I can from you about his needs."

Unless the person is a bully who routinely practices intimidating behavior (which we'll talk about later in this chapter), most people will realize that your intentions are good and regret their comment. It turns out that Margot had a very difficult shift and felt that she didn't give Mr. Jones the level of care she takes pride in delivering. When you asked all those questions, she thought you were insinuating that she didn't do a good job with her patient. Unwittingly, you contributed to the altercation by asking multiple questions. However, your choice to not respond emotionally and stay focused on the needs of the patient showed Margot that you weren't questioning her care. This helped get the interaction back on track.

"This experience taught me to persevere for the patient's well-being no matter how difficult the work environment may be." Suzette Cardin

Read Suzette's story, *Staying Positive Through Adversity*, on page 248.

What if You Choose Not to Respond? Is Silence Golden?

In the example above, we gave you only two choices – reacting negatively with anger and emotion or responding calmly and resolving the situation. There are, of course, other potential options. One of the most common is to stay silent and not take the chance of pressing the issue. This is often based on fear of eliciting a more negative and unpleasant response from the other person.

Yes a more unpleasant response is a possibility, but if you don't speak up, you have no chance of finding out what the real issue is – in this case, the other nurse thought you were questioning her nursing practice. The other danger of remaining silent is that you send the message that it's okay to treat you this way, which may invite future outbursts.

Remember, you're striving to know yourself better. If you don't think this is a good time to talk to the person because emotions are too high, then postpone the conversation for a time when you can discuss the issue calmly. But, you must follow-up as soon as possible.

Don't Stay Silent if Patient Safety is at Stake

If you're witnessing what you think is an error, omission or action that may cause a patient harm, then staying silent isn't an option.

In two studies, *Silence Kills* (2005) and *The Silent Treatment* (2010), conducted by the American Association of Critical Care Nurses and others, nurses remaining silent when witnessing an error, especially by an MD, occurs frequently and often results in catastrophic consequences for patients.

The 2005 study, *Silence Kills*, linked the failure of health professionals to discuss difficult topics with other health care team members, predominately physicians and nurses, to poorer patient safety and quality care outcomes and increased nursing staff turnover. Results indicated that only 10-12 percent of nurses participating in the study spoke up when they witnessed another's actions that could harm a patient.

A follow-up study in 2010, *Silent Treatment*, indicated that nurses' failure to speak up when they suspect an error or omission undermined the effectiveness of safety tools and procedures. Of the RNs participating in the study, 58 percent said that they failed to intervene because they felt their input would either be ignored or result in a negative outburst. The good news is that in the 2010 *Silent Treatment* study, the number of RNs who spoke up when patients were at risk increased to 21-31 percent as opposed to 10-12 percent in the 2005 study. Even though these numbers are increasing, there's still room for improvement.

Remember, you are the patient's advocate! You must speak up if you believe the actions of someone on the health care team may cause harm to a patient. If the person ignores you, call on the charge nurse or another colleague for help. To avoid future incidents, you may need to report and document the event.

Make Every Effort to Keep the Conversation Safe

In *Crucial Conversations*, Kerry Patterson et al., assert that difficult conversations often fail because one or both parties feel vulnerable and perceive that they're being attacked, blamed or put down. If a person in the conversation feels that way, it's highly unlikely they'll express their true feelings or concerns. Instead, they may lash out as a defense mechanism. The key to keeping the dialogue healthy or getting a derailed interaction back on track is to bring safety to the conversation.

You make the conversation safe by showing the other person that your goal isn't to attack or embarrass them, but to resolve the issue. They can tell you what they're thinking and feeling, and you'll listen. This doesn't mean you must agree with them – you still might not, but you're trying to understand where they're coming from and why they responded the way they did.

Let's look at an example:

You're a new grad in your fourth month on an oncology unit. You have a baccalaureate nursing degree, while most of the other nurses on your unit are prepared at the associate degree level. As part of your residency program, you're working on the floor as well as attending classes conducted by the hospital's clinical nurse specialists (CNS) and nurse educators. In a class you attended yesterday, a CNS covered the IV start protocol that the hospital has been following for approximately two years, and the reasons why it's a best practice.

"When we know in our hearts we're on the correct path – hold our heads high, shoulders back and march forward." Beth Gardner

Read Beth's story, *Dreams*, on page 274.

Today you observe Marti, one of the veteran nurses on the unit, using the old protocol which you know carries an increased risk of infection for the patient. You don't want to interrupt her during the procedure, but later you see her alone in the med room and decide to speak to her about it. The conversation goes something like this:

"Marti, Can I talk to you for a few minutes about the IV start on Mr. Johnson?"

"Of course. Do you want to run through the steps of starting an IV?"

"No, actually we covered IV starts in my new grad class yesterday. Janet, the CNS, gave us the newest protocol that was instituted two years ago in order to reduce IV infection rates. I was wondering if I could show it to you because you seemed to be following an older protocol when you started Mr. Johnson's IV."

You are surprised when Marti angrily responds:

"You new nurses think you know everything! I might not have a BSN, but I've been a nurse for 22 years and have started hundreds of IVs. And you think you can tell me how to do it better?"

You're stunned! Your intention was to be helpful. After all, the RNs on the floor have been giving you suggestions for months. Now you have something valuable to share that is safer for the patient, and Marti responds with anger.

One path you can choose is to respond with anger and emotion as well. "What's the matter with you! You won't even give me a chance to talk to you about something that's better for your patient! Do you treat everyone this way, or just me?" Or words to that effect. If this seems familiar – this is the path many would take. Perhaps you've taken this path before, too.

But pause for a moment and think about your goals. What do you want to achieve from this interaction? Your goals are to: prove yourself as an RN and contributing member of the team, improve patient care and safety on your unit and be accepted by your fellow nurses. Is an angry response going to help you get what you want?

Instead of reacting emotionally, you choose a different path. You take Marti's outburst as a sign that she doesn't feel safe. Maybe Marti thought you were putting her down with your comments, so she became defensive. Hopefully, you can get the conversation back on track by helping Marti feel safe again.

At this point you may be thinking: *Are you kidding? This person just yelled at me, and I should make them feel safe?*

We certainly don't condone these negative outbursts, but they do happen, and with some people, they may happen more frequently.

So if what you want is important to you, then yes, that's exactly what we're saying! We know it's not easy, but if you practice strategies for making and keeping your conversations safe for others, then you will be much more successful in your interactions and ultimately in achieving your goals.

Patterson recommends two approaches to keep conversations safe:

Mutual Purpose – Establish mutual purpose early in the conversation, for example: patient safety, the good of the team, creating a positive professional relationship, etc. By focusing on mutual purpose, it's easier to find common ground and avoid an offensive-defensive conversation, which is seldom productive. If the conversation starts to go awry, keep it on track by reminding the other person of your mutual purpose. If both of you can commit to a mutual purpose, you're well on your way to coming up with a beneficial solution.

Mutual Respect – There must be a level of mutual respect in order to have a chance at meaningful dialogue. Even if you choose your words carefully, a lack of respect can creep into your body language and/or tone of voice. You've probably seen it happen before – one person is trying to get their message across, and the other is rolling their eyes, shaking their head, not paying attention and/or using other negative body language.

Mutual respect can be difficult when you're having a conflict with someone because your focus is usually on the negative. You can build respect by keeping in mind the person's positive qualities. And yes, each and every person has some positive qualities. Maybe you want to talk with someone about their short, curt responses when you ask questions. Yet, you also recognize they have great technical skills – that's why you've been asking them questions in the first place. Perhaps, the nurse you frequently follow from the previous shift consistently fails to complete some tasks that then fall to you. However, you also recognize that this RN builds a wonderful rapport with her patients. By respecting these nurses' positive attributes, you can more positively focus on the negative behavior you want to discuss.

You may be thinking: *What about the other person? I want them to respect me in the conversation, too.* Unfortunately, you can't control someone else's behavior. You can only control yourself and model the type of behavior you'd like to see from the other party. If you remain calm, maintain your respect of the other person and stay focused on your mutual purpose, then hopefully the other person will feel safe in the conversation, see that you're sincere about working out the conflict and strive to reach a mutual solution.

Marti probably believes she is very skilled at starting IVs. If the new IV protocol has been in place for two years, then at some point, Marti probably rejected using it. Perhaps it was awkward at first and/or she didn't see the need to make the change (by the way, we'll talk about change and resistance to it in Chapter 7).

When you approached Marti about her IV start, she was getting ready to assume a teaching mode. She probably thought you were going to ask her questions about starting IVs in recognition of her skill. Marti may have viewed your suggestions as an attack on her abilities as a nurse. Her BSN comment could stem from a past conflict with a baccalaureate-prepared nurse, or her own regrets about not obtaining her BSN. We don't know if any or all of these possibilities are correct, but you can see some of the factors that might cause another person to react in a negative way. If you choose to take a productive path, rather than a destructive one, you can hopefully get the conversation back on track toward a positive outcome.

Building Mutual Purpose and Respect

We now know the importance of mutual purpose and respect, but how do we convey this to the other person in order to accomplish what we want out of the conversation? Here are some strategies Patterson recommends:

Apologize when appropriate – there are very few instances when one person is 100 percent wrong, and the other 100 percent right. Early in the conversation, admit your role in the issue or conflict, even if it's small. This will show the other person that you are sincere about resolving the problem, and aren't trying to affix blame on them. This may be difficult when you're in a conflict with someone. But once again, stay focused on what you want from the conversation.

After you've admitted your culpability, then hopefully the other person will be willing to admit theirs:

"Marti, I'm sorry if what I said made you think I'm questioning your skills as a nurse, that wasn't my intention. I think you're an excellent nurse – that's why I ask you so many questions."

In most instances, this will help the other person realize your intentions were good and bring safety to the conversation. Now you can continue with the issue:

"I didn't know if you were aware of this policy. Janet was very clear that research shows it's safer for the patients by reducing infection rates. I know how much you care about patient safety so I thought I'd share it with you."

"Although not all coworkers and bosses would be my best friends, I could work with them harmoniously by demonstrating competence, willingness to learn and professionalism." Kathy Cocking

Read Kathy's story, *Message on My Lunch Bag*, on page 252.

Contrast to Fix Misunderstanding

Even though you're trying to foster a level of mutual respect during the conversation, your words or actions may be misinterpreted by the other party. When that happens, don't ignore it, but instead address their feelings and the misunderstanding by using what Patterson calls contrasting. In contrasting, you utilize a *don't* and a *do* statement. The *don't* statement addresses the other person's concerns and the *do* statement clarifies your respect and/or mutual purpose. Then you can get back to the issue. Contrasting is not the same as apologizing. It's clarifying something you've said that the other person has misinterpreted, which is hindering your ability to reach a solution.

Don't statement: "Marti, I'm not trying to say I have all the answers."

Do statement: "You have a lot of knowledge and experience and you've really helped me grow as a new nurse."

Now, back to the business at hand:

"But Janet was very insistent that the new IV protocol is safer for the patients. Studies show it has significantly reduced IV infection rates. I shared it with you because I was trying to help you."

You can also use contrasting before you make a statement that you believe may cause defensiveness in the other person. This may head off a potential negative response before it even occurs. For example, you could have started the conversation with Marti like this:

"Marti, I learned some information in my class yesterday that I think you might be interested in. I know I'm not an expert in starting IVs – I've only started a few so far – but according to Janet, our CNS, the new IV protocol can help us reduce IV infection rates. Can I show it to you?"

By anticipating and responding first to potential problem areas in the conversation, you set the tone for a safe and productive dialogue. Hopefully, the other person will recognize this.

Agree on Your Mutual Purpose and Brainstorm Solutions

Why do you want what you're pushing for? Why does the other person? Once you've learned this information, you can discuss and agree on your mutual purpose. You may have the same purpose in mind, just different ideas about how to get there. Or, you both may have to adjust your purposes to incorporate each other's needs. Then you can brainstorm solutions that work for both of you.

Other Strategies to Keep the Conversation Productive

Don't Make Assumptions – A major cause of conflict and misunderstanding is when assumptions are made about what people did and why. Often, if someone doesn't have a complete picture of what happened, they make assumptions to fill in the blanks. Assumptions are based upon many of the concepts we talked about in the last chapter: personality, generation, culture, values, beliefs, etc. Often people will put more weight on the facts that support their assumptions, and ignore or minimize the facts that don't support them. This is human behavior – recognizing and addressing it is an important step in building good communication skills.

Instead of making assumptions, fill out the missing picture by asking questions and gathering more information. How many times have you observed others making assumptions about a situation you have firsthand knowledge of? You tell them what you observed, which is very different from the "story" floating around. Don't fall into this destructive trap. Until you've heard the full story, give others the benefit of the doubt.

Don't Generalize – Focus on the specific actions of the person you're talking to, don't generalize their behavior or actions by lumping them with others. For example: "Graduates from your school aren't good critical thinkers." Instead, focus on the individual and their actions or behavior.

Don't Talk in Absolutes – Absolutes, such as *always* or *never* hinder effective communication. With rare exception, no one always or never does or says something: you *always* yell at me; you're *never* nice to me; *no one* agrees with you. All the other person has to do is find one example to prove you wrong and you lose credibility.

Listen to the Other Person – When a conversation becomes heated, people often move into a competitive mode and strive to prove their position rather than seeking clarity and mutual agreement. While one person is talking, the other individual is focusing, not on what is being said, but instead on planning their response. If both parties are doing this, then they're talking at each other, without really listening. How much chance do you think they have of solving their issue?

If you want to have an effective conversation, then you must listen to what the other person is saying. Don't interrupt them. Focus on their words and body language. Try to show you're listening by using positive body language, such as nodding your head. If you don't understand something, ask a clarifying question when they finish their statement. When it's your turn to speak, if they interrupt you, then say: "Please let me finish." You can assess whether they understand what you're saying by asking questions.

Don't Take It Personally – As we discussed previously, a conversation can quickly escalate into conflict because one or both parties interpret a comment as a personal attack. Is it really an attack, or is the other person providing constructive feedback? If someone is giving you constructive feedback, then think about it in the spirit it was intended – to help you improve.

Even when someone acts out negatively, often the person who receives the brunt of their abuse isn't the intended recipient, but instead happened to be the unlucky one who approached this individual when they were in a highly stressed or foul mood. For example, some MDs have told us that when they've yelled at a nurse, it usually wasn't a problem with that particular nurse. Instead they were frustrated or angry about something else, and the nurse happened to ask them a question at that time. If a different nurse would have approached them at that moment, the reaction would have been the same.

Does this mean the outburst is acceptable behavior? Absolutely not! But if you realize that the behavior isn't aimed at you personally, it's much easier to deal with the situation calmly and objectively.

Call Timeout if the Conversation Gets Too Far Off Track – If the conversation becomes unproductive and/or hostile and there's no resolution in sight, then call a timeout. Both of you may need some time to think about the issues. If both parties think another meeting will help resolve the conflict – agree to meet at a future time. If you're at an impasse, consider involving an impartial third party to help the two of you settle the disagreement.

What About Difficult Conversations with Physicians?

The basic principles we discuss throughout this chapter are definitely applicable in conversations with physicians. However, MDs often won't invest too much of their time discussing an issue. Therefore, your window of opportunity is usually much shorter than a conversation with a fellow staff member. But you can still utilize the positive communication strategies we've described to help you accomplish your goals.

Here's an example:

Your 2nd-day post-op patient is complaining of significant pain. The oral pain medication he's receiving is not alleviating his discomfort. You approach his physician, who is sitting at the nurse's station, to report the patient's status and request stronger medication. Raising his voice, the doctor says: "Are you trying to kill my patient?" You're immediately embarrassed and feel your cheeks burning. But you take a deep breath and calmly reply: "Of course not. And he's my patient, too. I want what's best for him." A brief silence follows. The physician's anger diffuses, and the two of you discuss how to better control the patient's pain. Additional pain medication is ordered and safely administered to the patient.

This brief encounter illustrates using positive communication to diffuse conflict (by remaining calm, yet persistent), keeping the conversation productive (by establishing mutual purpose – the good of the patient) and achieving your ultimate goal (obtaining more effective pain medication for your patient).

Other strategies for communicating with physicians:

• Use data to make your case. Vital signs, intake and output, lab results and other objective facts are much more persuasive than feelings and emotions.

• Remain calm and professional, even if the physician is angry or emotional. This is tough to do, but will promote more effective communication. This doesn't mean you have to put up with abuse. It's okay to say: "Please don't speak to me that way. I have questions about Mr. Smith's care that we need to discuss."

• When pointing out an error, try to be as non-threatening as possible. Some strategies can include asking questions, comparing data and whenever possible, not calling attention to the error in front of others. For example:

"Dr. Smith, I'm just clarifying that Mr. Jones should receive 15 mg of Coumadin. He said at home he takes 5 mg daily."

"Dr. Mason, before I administer this IV potassium, let me show you Mrs. Brown's latest renal panel."

• If applicable, quote unit standards. "Dr. Allen, I can't administer that IV push medication because our unit standard prohibits it. For the safety of the patient, this drug must be administered by a physician or in a critical care area."

• Be persistent. Always remember you're the patient's advocate. If you believe the physician is about to make an error or isn't listening to your requests for something the patient needs, don't give up. If necessary, get your charge nurse, the department manager and/or the unit's medical director involved.

Giving and Receiving Feedback

Feedback is essential for us to grow personally and professionally. Receiving compliments and praise is easy and rewarding. But it's often difficult for people to hear about something they could have done better. Yet, it's our responsibility as professionals to provide constructive feedback to fellow team members to help them improve their expertise and skills. Giving feedback is a skill that improves with planning and practice.

These tips will help you provide appropriate feedback to your colleagues:

• Utilize the strategies we discussed earlier in this chapter about *Setting the Stage for Your Conversation.*

• Start with the positive and then go to the area that needs improvement.

• Focus on the incident or behavior, not on the person.

• Discuss one area of improvement at a time. Giving someone a laundry list of things to improve is confusing and likely to elicit a negative response. Stick to one issue and save the others for another time.

• Be specific – describe what the person did that was positive or caused a problem.

• Be timely – feedback is most effective when delivered as close to the event as possible. However, if there is too much emotion related to the situation, it's often better to wait until emotions are under control.

• Offer suggestions for improvement.

• Follow-up if needed.

If you are receiving feedback from someone else:

• Listen to what your colleague is telling you.

• Keep your emotions in check.

• If necessary, ask questions to clarify.

• Thank them for providing feedback, even if you don't agree.

• Think about how you can use this information to improve.

Bullying in the Workplace

"Bullying violates the ethical principle that is paramount to nursing – to respect the worth, dignity and human rights of all individuals – including colleagues." American Nurses Association

The word *bully* often conjures up images of a big, mean, aggressive kid in the schoolyard tormenting smaller children. Someone who spews forth physical and/or verbal abuse in order to instill fear in others – and seems to enjoy it. Unfortunately, bullying isn't confined to childhood or the schoolyard. It is a real and prevalent problem in many workplaces, and health care is no exception.

Some sources use disruptive behavior and bullying as interchangeable terms. It's important to distinguish that not everyone who exhibits disruptive behavior is a bully. However, all bullies exhibit disruptive behavior. As mentioned previously, many of us can and have exhibited disruptive behavior on occasion, often due to stress or other factors. Most of us are remorseful for our behavior. Bullies are not remorseful.

Sam Horn, author of the book *Take the Bully by the Horns*, defines a bully as:

"Someone who knowingly abuses the rights of others to gain control of a situation and the individual(s) involved. Bullies deliberately and persistently use intimidation and manipulation to get their way."

The key words in this definition that distinguish bullying behavior are: *knowingly*, *deliberately* and *persistently*.

Why do some people bully others? Common motivations for bullies are to:

- Call attention to themselves
- Control others
- Gain favorable assignments or reduced workload
- Feel better about their own shortcomings and insecurities
- Emulate behavior they've experienced – this is the way they were treated in the past, and they don't know any other way
- Test the boundaries to see how much they can get away with

Additionally, bullies are seldom remorseful for their actions. And because many receive no negative consequences for their behavior, they see no reason to change.

Let's look at some examples:

Scenario 1

Karen, a competent and conscientious RN, works on a cardiac telemetry floor. Dr. Logan, a cardiologist, is well known by nurses for badgering RNs he doesn't think measure up to his standards.

Other nurses on the unit advised Karen that in order to have a positive relationship with Dr. Logan, she needed to be more assertive and confident when communicating with him. If he became angry at her, Karen's coworkers advised that she must stand her ground and show him that she isn't afraid of him. This was his "test."

Karen, however, didn't pass Dr. Logan's test. Although she was a highly competent RN, whenever she spoke to him about a patient, she became nervous and tongue-tied. As a result, he would often verbally pounce on her. Each morning, she begged and bargained with other nurses to telephone Dr. Logan to report abnormal lab results for his patients so that she wouldn't have to do it. Nurse after nurse counseled Karen to be assertive when talking him. Some even role-played with her so that she could practice before speaking to him. But each time, she would again be overcome with nerves and fear. And again Dr. Logan would belittle her.

Eventually the situation got better as Karen slowly developed a more positive relationship with Dr. Logan. But because it took several months for Karen to assert herself, she suffered from his bullying for quite some time. And even though the situation improved, discussing a patient's condition with Dr. Logan still gives her butterflies.

From this scenario, there's no clear reason why Dr. Logan bullied Karen. It could be one or more factors, such as the need to control those caring for his patients, to call attention to himself, to test boundaries or some other combination of factors we don't know about. Sometimes the motivation isn't always clear.

Here's an example where the motivation is much more apparent:

Scenario 2

RN Kim would often have a verbal outburst when assigned a patient admit. She would angrily and loudly complain that she was being assigned the patient because the charge nurse didn't like her. Kim utilized this tactic with several charge nurses. Consequently, whether intentionally or not, some charge nurses were hesitant to assign new patients to Kim. Regardless of workload, they gave new patients to other RNs and only assigned Kim new admits as a last resort.

In this scenario, Kim's bullying and verbal abuse served her well – she often had a lighter patient assignment than other RNs on the unit. And since there were no negative consequences for her behavior, Kim continued to follow this pattern.

How Do You Stop the Bullying?

Whether or not the motivation is clear, bullying is unacceptable behavior and must be addressed.

According to Sam Horn, traditional communication methods usually don't work on bullies, often because they're not interested in resolving the situation or coming to a mutually beneficial agreement. The only interactions true bullies are interested in are ones that benefit them. They don't look for win-win opportunities, but instead try to manipulate the situation so that there is a winner and a loser – with them being the winners. Therefore, the first step is to determine if this person is truly a bully.

Remember, not everyone who exhibits difficult, disruptive or even bullying behavior on occasion is a true bully. As we stated previously, some people are mortified to learn that their conduct is considered disruptive or bullying. They're remorseful and take steps to modify their behavior. A true bully knowingly, deliberately and persistently uses intimidation and manipulation to get what they want at the expense of others. And they're *not* remorseful for their behavior or actions.

Is this Person a Bully?

• Does their negative behavior occur consistently and often?

• Have your attempts at trying to talk to them using positive communication techniques (as described earlier in this chapter) been shut down or thwarted by them? Or made the situation worse?

• Do you experience physical symptoms before, during and/or after interacting with them? For example, nervousness, digestive issues, sleeplessness, teeth grinding?

• Do you avoid them whenever possible?

• Do you walk on eggshells around this person, hoping that you're quiet enough or passive enough to get by them unscathed?

The sad truth about bullies is that they will often pick on someone they perceive as weaker, and therefore an easy mark. This can be a new graduate, a new employee, a staff member who is shy, someone from another culture, and the list goes on. Or, a group of two or more people may bully a single individual.

Regain Control: Don't Be a Target

Recognize that you are being bullied by this individual or group. Realize that you are not the cause of the problem – the bully is the source of these negative circumstances. It often has nothing to do with your skills, performance or actions. Once you truly realize that you're not the problem, you can begin to take control of the situation and your reactions to it.

If you've ever observed or perhaps been a victim of bullying behavior, you may wonder: *Why are there some people the bully never hassles?* The answer is that bullies often will only harass those they think won't challenge them or their behavior. They usually don't try their antics on someone they think will stand up to them. Bullying expert Sam Horn explains:

"Some people who act objectionably are in a way testing you to see what they can get away with. That's why it's so important to establish and enforce boundaries."

One way to minimize your chances of being bullied is to carry yourself so that you don't appear to be an easy target. This is one of the first skills taught in self-defense classes.

Don't Be a Target:

- Don't try to avoid the person who's harassing you – A bully will notice you're avoiding them and take this as a sign of weakness.
- Make direct eye contact when speaking with them – Avoiding their gaze, and looking down or away can be perceived as fear or weakness.
- When standing, stand upright and straight, on both feet with shoulders back and chest out.
- Walk purposefully, rather than hesitantly.
- Lean toward the person, instead of away.
- If you're sitting and they're standing over you exhibiting aggressive behavior, stand up and continue the conversation face to face.
- If the person steps into your personal space, don't step back, but instead stand your ground.

This body language will help you convey confidence and be less of a target for workplace bullying. You may be thinking: *I don't feel confident around this person – I feel nervous and hesitant.* Even if you're not feeling confident, train yourself to use more assertive body language. Practice in front of a mirror to see how the difference in your body language makes you appear more assertive. Even if you don't feel it right away, your body will convey confidence, which will in turn help you build more self-assurance.

Social psychologist Amy Cuddy has conducted several studies on nonverbal behavior and the origins and outcomes of how individuals are perceived by others. Her results indicate that when faced with an aggressive or dominant person, an individual will often assume a non-dominant or defensive posture and demeanor, which includes using closed body language, looking down or away from the person and making yourself smaller. This invites the aggressor to take control of the situation.

By displaying more powerful and assertive body language, you can discourage this aggressive behavior. Furthermore, Cuddy's research has shown that over time individuals displaying more powerful body language will produce higher levels of testosterone and decreased levels of cortisol, which lead to feelings of increased confidence and self-assurance. Therefore, if you practice more assertive body language, your feelings of confidence will catch up with your actions.

What Else Can You Do?

Don't suffer in silence. If attempts to deal with this issue haven't improved the situation, or have made it worse, here are some other strategies you can use:

• Refer to your organization's policies about bullying and disruptive behavior. It's a Joint Commission standard that hospitals have policies in place to address disruptive behavior. See if there are specific steps outlined in these policies you can utilize.

• Document the occurrences – Include dates, times, who else was present, what was said and done; how this impacted you, your ability to do your job and the effect on patient care. When you have enough data, talk to your supervisor or manager. If others complain of bullying or disruptive behavior, encourage them to also document and report the occurrences affecting them. It's very possible that the bully will deny or deflect your allegations. Documentation and other witnesses will help strengthen your position.

• Make sure your supervisor/manager understands the extent of the problem. Sometimes physicians or employees have exhibited bullying behavior for so long, that it's tolerated and ignored. Watch for phrases like: "Oh he's always like that, don't let it bother you." "She's a great nurse, she doesn't mean anything by it."

Be sure to emphasize how the behavior is affecting you, your team and/or patient care. If you're talking to your supervisor, and you don't believe they're going to address the issue, then you may need to take it up with the department manager. If you don't believe the manager will address these issues, consider reporting the behavior to your human resources department. As stated previously, your organization's policy on disruptive behavior can help guide your actions.

• Ask your manager for suggestions about how to deal with this person. Many managers will offer communication strategies and even role play with employees to help coach them through difficult communication situations with team members, MDs and/or patients and their families.

• Support others who are being bullied. Even though you're not the target, calmly interjecting a comment into a disruptive situation shows the disruptive person that their bad behavior is noticed by others and is not appropriate. For example:

"Sally, I'm not sure you realize it, but your voice is carrying and you sound really angry. Is there something I can do to help?"

Or:

"Dr. Smith, Sue is asking you questions to clarify your orders so there won't be any mistakes. Our goal is always to provide the best possible care and safety for the patients on this unit."

• Don't be discouraged if you don't see an immediate behavior change. If this is the first complaint about a staff member, the manager will need to investigate and gather more information about the employee and their behavior. If it's a physician, the issue must go through the medical staff channels.

YOU Can Make a Difference!

Confronting disruptive behavior and bullying can be difficult. But by using positive communication strategies, you can often improve the situation. According to the *Silence Kills* study we referred to earlier in this chapter, nurses who were confident in their communication skills and spoke up about patient safety issues, potential errors and disruptive behavior, achieved positive outcomes for their patients, their hospitals and themselves.

Becoming a skilled communicator doesn't happen overnight – it takes time and practice. Continue to read books and articles about building your communication skills. You can start with the resources on our reference list on page 287. Practice these methods to build your skills. Start with some "small" conversations. Evaluate your dialogue with others and look for ways to improve.

Although you won't be successful in every situation and some conversations won't go exactly as you'd like them to, you'll notice improved results. As you continue to practice, your confidence will grow and you'll feel satisfaction from being better able to handle difficult conversations and situations. You may even inspire others to speak up rather than suffer in silence.

You can make a difference – one conversation at a time!

Questions for Reflection

1. Have you ever seen colleagues make mistakes, circumvent practice standards or demonstrate serious incompetence?
    a. Did you speak up?
    b. If not, why not?
    c. What would help you feel comfortable to say something to them if you see this behavior again?

2. Have you ever felt that someone in the workplace has been condescending, insulting or rude to you?
    a. How does this behavior make you feel?
    b. Does this behavior affect your ability to perform your duties?
    c. How can you address this behavior when it happens again?
    d. What if this person is a physician?

Practice Scenarios

1. Your patient's potassium level is at the top of the normal range. Her physician just discontinued her diuretic but did not d/c her daily potassium supplements. You don't know if the MD saw the patient's labs and you're uncomfortable continuing to give potassium in this situation. What can you say to the physician?

2. You're a new hire nurse on a busy med/surg floor. You're assisting a nurse who has worked on the unit for several years. She is placing a Foley catheter in an elderly female patient. After putting on sterile gloves, the nurse adjusts her glasses and touches the bed. You point out to the nurse that her gloves are no longer sterile and offer to get her another pair. She laughs and says: "I'm just fine. Let's get this done – I have a lot of patients to see." What should you do?

3. You work on a unit with a group of staff members from another culture. This group of nurses often have conversations in their native language at the nurse's station and over patients. You feel uncomfortable because you don't understand what they're saying and you're afraid they're speaking negatively about you and/or the patients. What should you do?

4. You are an RN on a telemetry unit. The patient you've been taking care of for the past several hours has developed atypical chest pain with EKG changes. The physician has ordered that the patient be transferred to the ICU and a Nitro drip started. You accompany the patient to the ICU. When giving report to the patient's new nurse, you're about to stress the atypical symptoms of his chest pain. The receiving RN doesn't appear to be listening to you. She says: "We'll take it from here. I can get the information I need from the chart." You are concerned that the patient's atypical symptoms of chest pain may go unrecognized. What should you say to the ICU RN?

5. You are a new nurse in the emergency department. A woman brings her 80 year old mother to the ED. The patient has a headache, a temp of 101 and is very confused. Her daughter tells you that her mother is normally alert and oriented. According to the daughter, her mother displayed similar symptoms two years ago when she had meningitis. You place the patient in a room and ask the physician to see her right away. The physician's response is: "Another old lady who's confused – that's not an emergency. I'll see her later." When you try to discuss the matter further, he raises his voice and says: "I told you I'll see her later." What should you say to the physician?

Delegation: Empowerment and Accountability 6

"I attribute my success to this – I never gave or took any excuse."
Florence Nightingale

Today's health care leaders face the challenge of providing high quality patient care at a reasonable cost. A key strategy in balancing the complexity of health care with its cost is to identify and utilize the appropriate mix of personnel when designing care delivery systems. As registered nurses we play a key role, not only in providing direct patient care, but in assigning or delegating aspects of the patient's plan of care to other licensed and unlicensed members of the health care team. Your ability to effectively delegate has a strong impact on clinical outcomes and the quality of care for your patients.

Delegation is one of the most complex skills for new graduates to master. Although you were exposed to delegation theory in nursing school, your opportunity to practice these skills was most likely limited to the controlled environment of the simulation lab.

Now you'll be practicing the art of delegation in the clinical setting. Like many skills, effective delegation is learned through experience over time. This chapter will ground you in the important aspects of delegation as you build and refine your expertise.

What is Delegation?

The American Nurses Association (ANA) defines delegation as "the transfer of responsibility for the performance of a task from one individual to another while retaining accountability for the outcome." We delegate a task but *not* our accountability in the overall nursing plan of care.

Your state's *Nurse Practice Act* provides your authority to delegate. ANA's *Standards of Practice* describes our "responsibility for resource utilization, financial and human, when planning safe effective care." Furthermore, the ANA *Code of Ethics* offers clarity for our professional obligation in delegation: "The nurse is responsible and accountable for individual nursing practice and determines the appropriate delegation of tasks consistent with the nurse's obligation to provide optimum patient care." Finally, your employer's facility-specific policies and job descriptions provide the framework to actualize your authority to delegate in your work setting.

Learning to Delegate as a New RN

Pat shares this story:

I had the privilege of working as a nursing assistant the summer between my third and fourth semesters of nursing school, and spent several weeks on the medical floor. Following graduation, I was hired as an RN by this same hospital.

When I floated to the medical floor, I knew I would be working with staff members who had oriented me as a nursing assistant. Suddenly, this "kid" of 20 was supervising CNAs who had been providing direct patient care for 25 years. Early in the shift, I was struggling – trying to do my assessments, pass medications, superimpose IVs while also answering call lights and providing direct care. My stress level was almost through the ceiling when I felt a tap on my shoulder. The CNA who had oriented me over the summer quietly walked up behind me and said, "You're doing my job, delegate this to me."

This was the tipping point for me as I decided that if I was going to write RN after my name, I must embrace my role, including learning how and when to delegate.

Delegation Guidelines

Effective delegation requires an understanding of your professional authority and accountability, as well as knowledge of the role and scope of practice of those performing the tasks you delegate.

Transitioning into your new RN role is the perfect time to discuss delegation strategies and guidelines with your preceptor and nursing supervisor. Seasoned nurses are also excellent resources as you begin your journey to be an effective delegator. Talk to other experienced nurses about delegating practices.

Here are some suggested questions to get the conversation started:

- What type of tasks do RNs on this unit typically delegate to other members of the team?

- Which policies should I review to help me understand our unit's and hospital's philosophy of delegation?

- What resources are available on the unit and/or in the education department to assist me in understanding my role and responsibility in delegation?

- Does the hospital have a simulation lab where I can practice delegation in a controlled environment?

- How do I know if the unlicensed assistive personnel (UAPs) are competent?

- If I don't think a UAP is competent, what should I do?

- Can you share with me your favorite delegation story? What was your key learning?

These conversations can occur over several months as you grow in your RN role. As you listen to other nurses' experiences, think about how you can use this information to inform your practice. You'll soon discover that most experienced nurses continue to refine their delegation techniques throughout their careers.

Delegating Effectively

Clinical judgment and excellent communication skills are essential components of effective delegation. Your ability to successfully communicate with others is critical when delegating. Is your message clear? Was it understood by the receiver? Are you listening to any concerns they have after performing the task? When an error or poor outcome occurs related to delegation, it is often caused by ineffective communication or misunderstanding of the messages between the delegator and delegatee.

As a new nurse, you may experience conflicts or challenges when assigning or delegating activities to experienced licensed, certified and unlicensed members of the nursing team. Some of these individuals will test you to ascertain if you know your practice and the limits of theirs. But remember, you have the authority and responsibility by professional licensure to delegate to members of the team. Stay focused, calm and professional.

Use the key communication and conflict resolution strategies from Chapters 4 and 5 to navigate potentially difficult conversations. Your confidence as a communicator will lead to your competence in delegating. Always keep in mind that you are delegating tasks or aspects of the plan of care. You're not delegating the nursing process. As a professional, you retain responsibility for evaluating the outcome of the activities you delegate.

Our next section, *The Five Rights of Effective Delegation*, is an excellent tool to assist you when delegating to others.

The Five Rights of Effective Delegation

To guide nurses in delegating appropriately and successfully, ANA and the National Council of State Boards of Nursing (NCSBN) identify *Five Rights of Effective Delegation*. These five rights are a simple way to remember the key steps to consider when delegating.

Right Task – Select the appropriate tasks to delegate. You must determine what aspects of care can be safely and appropriately delegated. Years of experience and "other RNs let me do this…" doesn't make a delegated task right or legal. If you're not sure, check with your preceptor, supervisor or the facility's policies before you delegate a specific task.

Right Circumstance – Consider the overall needs of your patient. If you're going into a room to administer a patient's new antihypertensive medication, you should check the patient's blood pressure yourself. However, if the same patient needs their BP checked one hour later, and you know you'll be in the middle of a sterile dressing change, delegate checking the patient's vitals to a UAP (unlicensed assistive personnel), with clear direction that they're to report the results to you immediately if the patient's BP is outside the parameters you set for the patient.

Right Person – Select the right member of the team. Consider who on the team can carry out the task based on job description, scope of licensure, experience and competence. Perhaps a team member has a particularly good relationship with the patient or has additional expertise in caring for that patient population.

Right Directions – keep it simple and direct. Clearly communicate what you are delegating, the outcome you expect from completion of the task and the mechanism for providing you with feedback. It's your responsibility to ensure that the team member understands your communication. Encourage them to ask questions so they're clear about their responsibility related to the delegated task. If necessary, ask the team member to repeat back what they'll be doing and their responsibility in providing you with information after completion of the task.

Although you want to keep your instructions simple, providing additional information about the importance of the task can be a motivator for the team member who will be completing it. For example: "Please take Mr. Smith's blood pressure in one hour, and report back to me if the systolic is below 100 or diastolic is below 60. He just started a new med, and I want to make sure it doesn't cause his BP to drop too low."

"That night I learned that I needed to listen - really listen - to members of my team and 'hear' what they were telling me."

Peggy Diller

Read Peggy's story, *The Art of Listening*, on page 246.

Right Supervision – The oversight and evaluation phase of delegation is as important as the task itself. Don't assume that because you delegated a task, it was carried out. You must follow up with the team member and the patient. Key questions you may ask the team member include: How did the patient tolerate the activity? Did you observe anything that was unusual or different from your previous interactions with the patient? Do you have any concerns about the patient? By asking for the team member's observations and concerns, you're demonstrating an appreciation of their contribution to the care of the patient, while at the same time ensuring that the task was completed. Effective communication includes listening as well as speaking.

Effective Delegation Includes Listening

Pat shares this story:

While working as the charge nurse in a 10-bed ICU, I was asked to float Marge, our unit's LVN, to the pediatric department. The nurses on our unit trusted Marge's judgment and valued her contributions to the care of our critically ill patients. She was very competent with more than 10 years of clinical experience. When we were new graduates, Marge helped us learn how to delegate effectively and, more importantly, how to value the contributions of all team members.

About two hours into the shift, Marge called our unit asking to speak with me. She shared her concerns about a newly admitted 9-month old patient. I reminded Marge that she must discuss this with the pediatric staff and the RN she was assigned to work with. After some coaching, Marge agreed to approach the staff again to share her concerns. About 10 minutes later, Marge was on the phone again, asking me to come to the peds floor. I knew by her tone of voice and insistence that I should stop what I was doing and go assess the situation. When I arrived, I immediately recognized that her young patient was in respiratory distress. I alerted the RN assigned to the patient and the house physician. Within minutes the child was intubated and transferred to the ICU.

This was a situation where the RN had delegated the task of monitoring this child's vital signs every 15 minutes to Marge, an LVN. Marge carried out the task as directed. She understood her scope of practice, and attempted to provide the RN with the critical data she was collecting about the child. Marge recognized the change in the patient's condition, and knew her responsibility was to inform the RN. The RN was at fault for failing to listen to her.

To this day, I believe Marge saved this patient's life. Had she not been persistent about reporting her findings to an RN, the child most likely would have suffered dire consequences.

In Summary – Key Delegation Reminders

• As the registered nurse, you are delegating the task or specific aspect of care to a qualified, competent member of the health care team. You are *not* delegating your authority or responsibility for the nursing process.

• Delegation is a professional behavior that gets easier as you become more confident and competent in your professional role.

• If at any point you feel that delegating a task isn't in the best interest of the patient, then don't delegate it! Share your concerns with your preceptor, supervisor or a senior staff nurse to gain insight into the situation.

• Always use the *Five Rights of Delegation* to guide you.

• Effective communication and listening are key elements for successful delegation.

• Be open to strategies for improving your delegation and communication skills.

• Mastering delegation is a major component of professional excellence.

• When delegating, it is imperative that RNs know their state-specific practice act and accompanying rules and regulations, as well as their employer-specific policies and procedures related to delegation.

Delegation is more than simply assigning tasks to members of the health care team. When delegation is based on a checklist of tasks, rather than patients' needs, patient safety and quality of care are compromised. When professional decision-making is utilized, tasks are delegated by matching the needs of the patient with the competence and experience of team members. Capitalizing on each staff member's unique contributions and expertise is essential for effective delegation.

As you grow to appreciate the depth and breadth of your practice accountabilities and responsibilities, you'll begin to understand your role in delegation. Learning to effectively delegate enables nurses to coordinate care to meet the complex health needs of their patients. As your confidence and skills grow, you'll see that effective delegation benefits you, the health care team and above all, your patients.

Questions for Reflection

1. Observe your preceptor or another senior nurse as they delegate a task to a staff member. Did they follow the *Five Rights of Delegation*? How was the delegation received by the other staff member? What, if anything, would you have done differently in this delegation scenario? What learnings did you gain from this observation?

Practice Scenarios

1. Your patient needs a chest tube. The physician is coming to the unit in 30 minutes to insert the chest tube. Your preceptor has helped you gather the supplies and then delegated to you the task of assisting the physician. You have never seen or helped with a chest tube insertion. How would you handle this situation? What are your resources? How can you turn this situation into a positive learning experience?

2. You have an LVN/LPN and a UAP working with you. The shift is very busy. Twice you've tried to connect with the LVN/LPN to discuss the status of two of the patients she's been caring for. She tells you that she's too busy to talk and not to worry because she has everything under control. What should you do?

Opportunity or Uncertainty: Successfully Managing Change

"You must be the change you wish to see in the world."
Mahatma Gandhi

Change plays a significant role in your professional and personal life. It can result in tremendous opportunity, great turmoil – or both. It can leave you disoriented, apprehensive and uncomfortable, even if you recognize and welcome the need for change.

The rate of change in our organizations and lives is growing at a rapid pace. Harvard professor, author and change guru John Kotter explains:

"By any objective measure, the amount of significant, often traumatic change in organizations has grown over the past two decades. Powerful macroeconomic forces are at work here, and these forces will grow even stronger over the next few decades. As a result, more and more organizations will be pushed to reduce costs, improve the quality of products and services, locate new opportunities for growth and increase productivity."

Health care is no exception. Over the past few years, we've seen tremendous change in patient care delivery, technology and regulatory requirements. As patients utilize the Internet and social media to select their hospitals and care providers, the vast majority of health care organizations are continually striving to improve patient safety, quality of care and customer service. The drive to improve services, while reducing costs, has resulted in tremendous change in relatively short periods of time.

As new grads, you're experiencing significant change as you transition from nursing student to staff nurse. Such rapid change can elicit feelings of doubt, discomfort, inadequacy and fear of failure. Understanding how you react to change is the first critical step in successfully managing change in your life and seizing the opportunities and rewards change can bring.

Our Reaction to Change

After spending several years in large health care organizations, your authors have seen several change initiatives come and go, and many frustrated managers and administrators wringing their hands saying: "It's not that difficult! Why don't they just do it?"

Unfortunately, human behavior isn't often that simple!

In his book, *Transitions*, psychologist William Bridges describes three phases we experience when we go through significant change. Understanding these three phases and the resulting reactions to them, can help you effectively cope with and manage changes in your life.

Phase 1: Endings

"What we call the beginning is often the end...The end is where we start from." T.S. Eliot

Any successful change first begins with an ending. The end of our existing way of doing something – whether it's a process, procedure, equipment, the management structure or a change in our job role. The change can be large or small, but it all begins with the end of something.

In a major change, you're not only leaving behind something, but also the meaning you derived from the previous way of doing things. You may have heard colleagues say: "This isn't why I became a nurse!" Struggling with major change can impact our identity.

Letting go can be difficult. But Bridges contends that you must deal with the ending before moving on to whatever is coming next. This ending can actually trigger a grief response. You grieve for what you lost or are about to lose.

Maybe you're getting a new boss – part of the apprehension you're feeling could be that you're grieving for the loss of the relationship with your old boss. Perhaps your job is changing, and you're worried that your new role won't give you the joy the old one did. You may be grieving the loss of those positive feelings in your life.

As you learned in nursing school, the grieving process, as described by Elisabeth Kubler-Ross, consists of five phases – anger, denial, bargaining, depression and finally acceptance. There's no time limit for how long it takes to pass through these stages, this varies by individual.

Some people will jump back and forth between these phases until they finally are in the acceptance phase and acknowledge and accept the loss. Others never accept the loss.

If you perceive that the change creates a loss for you, then you must let yourself grieve for this loss. By acknowledging your feelings, you can work through the grieving process and move forward.

Another source of stress in Bridges' *Ending Phase* is fear of the unknown – the uncertainty of the new state to be created by the change. This uncertainty often produces feelings of doubt. *Will I be happy in the new state? Will I be successful? What if I can't master the new skills I'm going to need?* The questions, fears and doubts about the unknown can be overwhelming and very unsettling.

Successfully Moving Through the *Ending Phase*

Recognize and acknowledge that the proposed change is going to bring about the end of "something." If this "something" is important to you, it may trigger the grieving process. Acknowledge your feelings and allow yourself to move through the stages of grief. Think about and, if necessary, make a list of what you'll lose with this change. Only when you have a clear picture of what is lost, can you begin the process of letting go.

Gather as much information about the change as possible. Do you know how the change will affect you? If you don't know, what can you do to find out? Lack of information is one of the major reasons people resist change and new initiatives fail.

Be careful about misinformation and the rumor mill. People who don't have all the facts about something often fill in the blanks with assumptions, speculation and/or past experiences. These are often inaccurate and can mushroom into clouds of misinformation about the upcoming change.

Possessing accurate, thorough information about the change will help you realistically assess how the change will affect you, and what the new state will be like. It will also help you determine how your skills will fit in the new state. Fear of the unknown can best be overcome by learning as much about the change as possible. The sooner you get accurate information about why the change is necessary and what the future vision is, the sooner you can move through the *Ending Phase*. To learn more about the change, talk to your manager, attend employee forums and read the employee newsletter or other sources of information about the upcoming change.

Recognize and celebrate what you've accomplished. Think about the approaching ending. Celebrate what you accomplished during the old way of doing things and start thinking about the possibilities of the new state. Just because a process or system is changing, this doesn't negate all the good work that came before. Take pride in your accomplishments related to the old system and recognize that the change is necessary to assure continued care, quality, service, etc.

Phase 2: The Neutral Zone

"It's not so much that we're afraid of change or so in love with the old ways, but it's that place in between that we fear." Marilyn Ferguson

Now that you've accepted that the old way is ending, you move into what Bridges calls the *Neutral Zone*. This is an in-between time, a transition between the old and new ways.

Although the *Neutral Zone* is a necessary phase in the change process, it can be extremely distressing. For many, this is a time of confusion and instability; a time of waiting and wondering. *Am I prepared for the new state? Will I be happy in the new system? Will I fit in?* You may experience a loss of control and purpose. Be assured – this is a natural phenomenon – one that Bridges says we all experience in times of change.

In this transition phase, you and/or some of your peers may still be grieving the loss of the old way. This is a critical time for implementation of the change. Because people will feel uncomfortable with the transition process, some may resist the change and try to revert to the old structure and familiar habits.

Communication between staff and leadership is vital in this phase. Communication should be two-way so that employees have the opportunity to vent their feelings about the change. If the leadership wants the change to be successful, then as much as possible, they should involve staff in planning and implementing the change.

In the *Neutral Zone* or transition period, you will often receive information, training and preparation to adapt to your new role, process or way of doing things. Information and knowledge about the new vision is especially important in the *Neutral Zone*. As you build your knowledge and skills for the new situation, you take back control of your professional life.

Seize this Opportunity to Build Your Skills

Think of this change and transition period as a time to update your skills and build new ones. A time to increase your knowledge base and expand your horizons.

Seizing the Opportunity to Add to Your Toolkit

Brenda shares this story:

In the mid-90s, our hospital was moving to a computerized order entry system. This was a major change and many were resistant. The organizational plan was to draft employees from various disciplines, such as nursing, pharmacy and lab, and teach them to be trainers and support staff for the implementation of this new system. The theory was that employees would be more open to receiving training from their peers, rather than consultants.

I saw this as an opportunity to get some experience as a trainer and see if I liked working in an educational setting, which was a career path I was considering. I was hired for one of the training slots (mainly because very few RNs applied) and given a nine-month leave of absence from my unit to work on the project.

The problem was, like many nurses at the time, my computer skills were practically nonexistent. Initially, we went through a two-week training period to learn the new system. On my first day of class, I embarrassingly had to ask how to turn on the computer. I later learned that many of my fellow trainers started their own classes by saying: "Don't worry, anyone can learn this system. We have a trainer who didn't even know how to turn on her computer the first day and now she's teaching classes!"

Through this nine-month stint as a computer trainer, I learned that I loved teaching others. It helped launch a very happy ten-year career as a hospital educator and later manager in the organization's staff development department. I may never have taken that plunge without my experience as a computer trainer.

As you move through the *Neutral Zone,* consider what opportunties there might be for you. How can you take control and make this a positive growth experience? Again, seek out as much information as you can about the change.

If you're learning new skills, your productivity will decrease as you update your knowledge and skill set. Don't be discouraged if and when this happens. Remember the novice to expert journey (Chapter 1) and your past successes in mastering other nursing skills. In time, any new skills you learn will become second nature.

Phase 3: The New Beginning

"You've gone through the first two phases of transition. Now you'll see that your New Beginning has been there with you for a while, waiting for you to notice." William Bridges, PhD

In this phase, you've moved through the *Neutral Zone* and are feeling at least somewhat comfortable in your new role or with the new process. As you continue to practice your new skills, your comfort and confidence will continue to grow. Organizationally, systems should be fully aligned with the change in order to prevent slippage back to the old ways.

Celebrate how far you've come and congratulate yourself for learning and utilizing new knowledge and skills. Hopefully, your leaders will also recognize what you and your colleagues have accomplished to get here.

At this point, Bridges recommends you take some time to re-examine the expectations and feelings you experienced during the *Ending Phase*. Were your original expectations and fears accurate? If yes, that's great! You probably have realistic expectations about change and how you react to it. If the answer is no, think about how your expectations and fears differed from reality.

Also, think about what phase was most difficult for you. Try to identify why. By analyzing your reactions to change, you can more effectively manage future changes in your life.

Has Everyone Adapted to the Change?

You may observe colleagues who are resistant throughout the change process, even as the new state is fully implemented and functional in your department and/or organization. Chances are, these folks never successfully moved from the first two phases in the change cycle. Perhaps they haven't successfully dealt with the *Ending* of the old way, or are stuck in the limbo of the *Neutral Zone*.

At times, staff members who have not yet accepted the change may try to disrupt the process by refusing to adapt and encouraging others to do the same. If you want to help them successfully acclimate to the change, assist them in seeing that the old way has ended and encourage them to face their feelings about this ending. Tell them what you know about the change – why it's necessary, how it will improve patient care, efficiency or whatever else it's designed to improve. Be sure to focus on the facts, not rumors. Encourage them to talk to their leaders about the change. Perhaps they need more information, additional training or assurance that they'll be able to adapt to the change and the new way of doing things.

What if You're Having Trouble Adapting to the Change?

Think about why this particular change is difficult for you. Is it because you don't want the current way of doing things to end? Perhaps you don't see how the change will be an improvement. Or maybe you believe the change conflicts with your values.

As we stated earlier in the chapter, one of the main reasons people don't accept a change is uncertainty due to lack of information. Discuss this with your preceptor, manager or someone else who can shed more light on the specifics of the change and the purpose behind it.

Suggestions to get the conversation started:

• I'm interested in learning more about this change. Here's what I know about it. Can you give me more information or direct me to resources so that I can learn more?

• How do you see this change improving patient care, our system (or whatever the change is supposed to improve)?

• Will there be training to help us adjust to the change? (Or if there has been training, perhaps you feel that you need more). I would feel more comfortable and confident if I had additional training. Can this be arranged?

As you use the new system or process, you may find problems that need to be addressed. When you become aware of issues or have suggestions for improvement, discuss these with your supervisor. Put your efforts into making the change positive by using it as a springboard for improvement.

"Change will not come if we wait for some other person or some other time. We are the ones we've been waiting for. We are the change that we seek!" President Barack Obama

Helping Your Patients Cope with Change

Illness can result in major lifestyle changes for our patients. As nurses, we sometimes have difficulty understanding why patients are resistant to changing their habits, especially when these changes promote optimal health.

While Bridges' model, discussed earlier in this chapter, provides an excellent framework to help you understand the feelings your patients may experience when coping with illness and resulting lifestyle changes, its application is better suited for long-term nurse-patient relationships. For many RNs, therapeutic encounters with patients are often short-term, especially in the acute care setting.

Kurt Lewin, a pioneer of change theory, developed a simple model that can be effectively applied by nurses to help their patients implement lifestyle changes. Lewin's theory of *Force Field Analysis* states that when an individual is faced with change, there are *Driving Forces* (positives supporting the change) and *Resisting Forces* (obstacles to change).

If the *Driving Forces* are greater than the *Resisting Forces*, the change will most likely occur. However, if the *Resisting Forces* are greater or equal to the *Driving Forces*, then the change effort will most likely fail (see *Force Field* diagrams on opposite page).

Sounds simple! Now let's take a look at how this can apply in the health care setting:

Mrs. B is a 75 year-old widow who lives alone. She has been hospitalized for uncontrolled hyperglycemia related to diabetes. Among other problems, her chronically uncontrolled blood sugar levels have resulted in retinopathy. Mrs. B's MD just broke the news to her that these visual changes mean she should no longer drive a car. Mrs. B's three adult children are worried that she won't accept this change and will drive despite her doctor's warning. As Mrs. B's nurse, you're preparing to educate her about healthier lifestyle choices and why she must heed the physician's warning to not drive.

In talking to Mrs. B and her family, you discover the following forces influencing this change:

Driving Forces for Mrs. B's Change

• Safety – if Mrs. B drives with her impaired vision, she's a danger to herself and others.

Resisting Forces Against Mrs. B's Change

• Loss of independence – If Mrs. B can't drive, how will she run

Lewin's Force Field Analysis

Driving Forces
Positive Forces for Change

Resisting Forces
Obstacles to Change

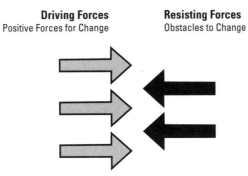

When the *Driving Forces* (forces supporting the change) are greater than the *Resisting Forces* (obstacles to change), the change will most likely occur.

Driving Forces
Positive Forces for Change

Resisting Forces
Obstacles to Change

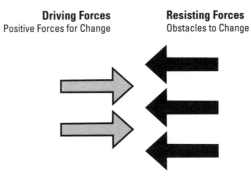

When the *Resisting Forces* are greater than the *Driving Forces*, the change effort will often **not** be successful.

Driving Forces
Positive Forces for Change

Resisting Forces
Obstacles to Change

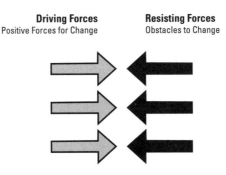

When the *Driving Forces* and the *Resisting Forces* are equal, the change effort will often **not** be successful.

errands, go grocery shopping, etc.? Is this just the first of other changes limiting her independence?

• Doesn't want to burden others – If Mrs. B can't drive, she's afraid her children will be forced to transport her. They do a lot for her already and she doesn't want to further infringe on their lives.

• Heightened awareness of her mortality – Underlying this change may be the fear that her diabetes will result in other negative health consequences and may ultimately result in her death.

• Driving is an activity she enjoys – Mrs. B genuinely likes to drive, and the thought of not being able to operate her car makes her sad and angry.

As an objective bystander, the decision may at first seem simple to you – Mrs. B should no longer drive her automobile because it's unsafe. But as you can see, there are several *Resisting Forces* influencing Mrs. B's decision about whether to stop driving her car. According to Lewin's theory, to help Mrs. B understand and accept this change, you must add to the *Driving Forces*, negate some of the *Resisting Forces* and/or convert a *Resisting Force* to a *Driving Force* supporting the change.

How can we do that? First let's look at the *Driving Forces*:

• Safety – People are often willing to accept some risk for themselves if they think the benefits outweigh the risks. However, they are averse to putting others in danger. As Mrs. B's nurse, you can stress that driving with her impaired vision could result in harm to others, especially pedestrians, bike riders and children – who are often more difficult to see when driving.

Additional *Driving Forces* Mrs. B may not have considered:

• Potential financial liability – Mrs. B could be liable for damages if she has a car accident and it's discovered that her doctor said she shouldn't drive.

• Increased anxiety for her family – If Mrs. B continues to drive, her children will worry about her safety.

Now let's look at the *Resisting Forces* that could be negated or converted to *Driving Forces*:

• Loss of independence – Mrs. B may not be aware of the services in her community, such as senior shuttles to the grocery store, *Meals on Wheels* and other assistance. In addition, many grocery stores deliver, she may be able to go shopping with a neighbor, or perhaps Mrs. *B* could hire a college student looking for extra cash to transport her. By utilizing other options, Mrs. *B* can maintain her independence.

• Doesn't want to burden others – Encourage Mrs. *B*'s children to discuss options with her. A weekly shopping trip could be a great outing for Mrs. *B* and one of her children. As noted previously, Mrs. *B* didn't consider how much her family would worry about her if she continues to drive. Not wanting to cause her family anxiety is an additional *Driving Force* for this change.

• Heightened awareness of her mortality – This is a common fear for seniors. In Mrs. *B*'s case, this fear has been amplified due to her uncontrolled diabetes. Give her an opportunity to talk about these fears, and provide teaching about healthier lifestyle options to better control her disease, minimize symptoms and maintain optimal health for her condition.

• Driving is an activity Mrs. *B* enjoys – As discussed earlier in this chapter, change often initially results in a loss. This loss can trigger a grief response. Allow Mrs. *B* the opportunity to grieve for the loss of her ability to drive. Educate her family about the grief process so they can support her as she makes this important change.

By acknowledging the driving and resisting forces for any given change, you can help your patients and their families better cope with the lifestyle changes that are often a result of illness and aging.

Take Control of the Change Process

"The door that nobody else will go in, seems always to swing open widely for me." Clara Barton

Change is a powerful influence in your career and personal life. It can be difficult and anxiety-provoking, especially if the change is unwanted. In this chapter, we've given you an overview of human responses to change and the forces that can drive change or resist it. By better understanding how people react to change, you can take control and create opportunities from the changes in your life, rather than passively riding the tide of change wherever it may take you.

Questions for Reflection

1. When you think of making a major change in your professional life, what feelings do you experience? Are they positive, such as excitement, anticipation, a sense of adventure? Or negative, such as fear, apprehension, uneasiness?

2. When considering Bridges' three phases of change, which phase is the easiest for you? Which is the most difficult?

Ending

Transition

New Beginning

What could you do to make the most difficult phase easier?

3. Think about a recent positive change you experienced. How did you feel making the change? Why was it positive? What did you learn about your response to change from the experience?

4. Think about a recent change that was difficult or not sustainable. Why do you think the change was so difficult? What did you feel during the process? What did you learn from the experience?

Quality and Patient Safety: You Can Make a Difference!

8

"Save one life and you're a hero. Save 100 lives and you're a nurse." Chuck Stepanek

Nurses have been on a journey to improve the quality of patient care since the days of Florence Nightingale. Nightingale was a visionary leader who recognized the importance of using data to improve care. Her interventions related to infection control, sanitation and nutrition greatly improved patient outcomes during the Crimean War and beyond. Her actions as a nurse saved countless lives.

Although in our current health care system we've been successful at implementing many quality improvement initiatives, thousands of patients continue to experience medical errors each year. Just like Florence Nightingale before us, nurses have a professional obligation to improve patient care by correcting systems or practices that place our patients at risk.

The quality movement is rapidly evolving based on new evidence. This makes it difficult to keep abreast of current recommendations and practices. The goal of this chapter is to provide you with an overview of the quality movement, key quality initiatives and a look at some of the entities at the forefront of the pursuit to improve patient safety and outcomes. We'll also discuss how you can positively impact the quality of care on your unit.

"The weighty responsibility of having a life entrusted into my care was indelibly etched in my heart and mind."
Gwen Matthews

Read Gwen's story, *Was I Never Meant to be a Nurse?*, on page 192.

The Quality Movement

"Quality health care is a human right for all. To improve the quality of care, health care professionals must address these complex issues: increasing costs of care, health disparities and the lack of safe accessible, and available health care services and resources."

ANA Social Policy Statement, 2010

Consumers, providers, insurers and regulators are demanding improvements in our health care system. Consumers today are more informed and educated about health and health care than ever before. They want improved access to personalized, quality care at a reasonable cost. Providers want to practice to the full extent of licensure without barriers restricting their ability to provide appropriate individualized care. Third party payers seek to control costs while ensuring their members have access to quality care. The government is mandating strategies to increase access, improve quality and decrease cost. The common denominator is the expectation for quality health care by the consumer, provider, purchaser and regulator.

At the advent of the quality movement, health care leaders looked to business, manufacturing and the airline industry for strategies to improve quality. At the time, business had embraced the work of W. Edwards Deming and his quality management principles, including the *Plan, Do, Check, Act* cycle. Later, other theorists including Cosby, Juran and Ishikawa added to Deming's work, and these combined philosophies are referred to as *Total Quality Management* (TQM).

TQM is a philosophy promoting excellence and improvement at all levels of an organization. Health care organizations adopting TQM principles are committed to removing barriers and empowering employees to identify and implement strategies leading to patient care improvements. TQM has been operationalized through quality improvement activities and continuous quality improvement (CQI) strategies.

For optimal results, it's essential that all members of the health care team embrace the CQI concept. Senior management must take responsibility for establishing the vision and environment for quality improvement activities to flourish. They must empower staff to look for and recommend ways to improve processes. Successful health care leaders have implemented programs to engage staff in quality improvement activities, including *Six Sigma, Lean, TeamSTEPPS* and other processes embracing rapid cycle change.

An excellent example of a highly successful, staff-driven quality improvement effort is the Transforming Care at the Bedside (TCAB) program. TCAB is a Robert Wood Johnson Foundation (RWJF) and Institute for Healthcare Improvement (IHI) collaborative project designed to improve the care patients receive on medical-surgical units. The TCAB framework for improvement is built around four main themes: safe and reliable care, vitality and teamwork, patient-centered care and value-added care processes. TCAB involves the entire team and is based on the premise that work redesign involves those closest to the issue. Empowered TCAB teams have the authority to execute change and implement systems leading to or resulting in improved outcomes. A number of outstanding processes have been designed and implemented by direct care staff involved in the TCAB project.

Of the many innovative programs generated through TCAB, one outstanding example is the concept of rapid response teams (RRT). The goal of the RRTs is to bring critical care expertise to the bedside of medical/surgical patients experiencing deterioration in their condition. In essence, the RRT "rescues" the patient before a crisis occurs. In this model, resources are made available to the staff in units outside the critical care setting so that critical care and med/surg nurses can work together to implement care processes and prevent further deterioration in the patient's condition.

Utilization of RRTs has not only improved the care provided to patients in facilities where this program has been implemented, but the increased communication between the staff has led to improved relationships, mutual respect, enhanced opportunities for learning and increased job satisfaction for those involved.

Asking the Question

Pat shares this story:

As a nursing director, I participated in extensive TQM/CQI training programs, and was a member of several teams working to improve the care processes in our hospital. We received recognition for our ventilator program years before the *Ventilator Acquired Pneumonia* (VAP) bundle was introduced by the Institute for Healthcare Improvement.

No matter what quality project we were working on, there was one question we learned to ask ourselves throughout the process: *"Ask the Clinicians!"* It affirmed the foundation of CQI principles – that leadership must remove the barriers to practice improvement – but it is the professionals closest to the issue who often have valuable insight into the problem and potential solutions. This mantra taught me to seek input and help from all those who would be affected by the change before initiating a change or implementing new projects. This is a valuable learning I continue to embrace today!

Just Culture

Historically, quality programs were about identifying errors, finding the person responsible and then blaming or punishing that individual for the mistake. Disciplining employees for unintentional human error doesn't promote an environment for patient safety, enable people to learn from mistakes or prevent future errors. Even the best clinicians can make mistakes – it's called being human.

Once it was recognized that trying to eradicate human error was impossible, the focus of the quality movement turned to the development of systems to catch or minimize errors before a patient is harmed. This shift in focus resulted in the utilization of the *Just Culture* concept.

Adopted from the airline industry, a *Just Culture* is a learning environment where errors are investigated and systems corrected in order to reduce future mistakes. It is important to remember that in a *Just Culture* environment, individuals retain accountability for their practice and adherence to the organization's clinical and practice standards. But by changing the focus of error prevention from blame and punishment to opportunities for learning and improvement, potentially harmful mistakes can be identified and significantly reduced. The only exception is when the error resulted from intentional negligence. Even in a *Just Culture*, errors made through intentional negligence often will result in disciplinary action.

A *Just Culture* looks at the choices the individual or team made in relation to the error. Did the person simply make the wrong choice or inadvertently do something that resulted in an error? Did they make a decision knowing it wasn't quite right but decided to risk the situation anyway? Did they know they were making a decision that was wrong, but simply didn't care?

In a *Just Culture*, the handling of errors is based on the choices or behaviors of the individuals involved. These behaviors fall into three categories:

Human Error – If the mistake is the result of a human error or inadvertent action, management will console the staff member while implementing strategies to ensure that the individual learns from the situation. The focus is on determining what systems can be initiated or improved to prevent or minimize this type of error in the future.

Example: Several unexpected events occurred during your shift and, as a result, you missed a dressing change for your patient. You notice this during rounds at the end of the shift. How can you change your system of managing tasks so that important treatments aren't missed in the future?

At Risk Behavior – If the staff member makes a choice that's considered a risk, the individual is coached regarding the potential consequences of the choice they made, as well as alternatives that increase safety for the patient.

Example: You've had a hectic day. At the end of your shift you remembered that you didn't empty your isolation patient's Foley bag. You know you're going right home after work, so you decide to run into the patient's room and empty the Foley without putting on a gown and mask. Your manager is standing in the hallway and notices you've failed to take proper precautions. Your failure to follow hospital policy on isolation has put you, your peers and patients at risk. What strategies would you adopt to prevent this from happening in the future?

Reckless Behaviors – The staff member's actions exhibit a conscious disregard for the standard of care resulting in an unjustifiable risk to patient safety. Even in a *Just Culture*, this behavior results in disciplinary action because it wasn't human error, but an intentional act.

Example: You receive a transfer patient from the ICU, who is receiving a blood transfusion. As you're receiving report and checking documentation, you notice there's only one signature (that of the RN transferring the patient to you) verifying that the blood product is correct. When you point this out to the RN, he says: "We know what we're doing! We don't need another person to check with us."

This RN is putting his patient in grave and unnecessary risk by intentionally circumventing a standard of care proven to reduce blood administration errors.

Through *Just Culture*, many health care organizations strive to create non-punitive, fair environments. In a *Just Culture*, staff members accept personal and professional accountability for practice and actively work collaboratively to improve the processes of care by focusing on learning and building improved systems.

"I received the support I needed. I was consoled by my manager, but I was also accountable for my actions."
Robyn Nelson

Read Robyn's story, *Was It Early Just Culture?*, on page 234.

Learning from a Medication Error

Brenda shares this story:

I had been a nurse for about a year on the12-hour night shift of an interventional cardiology unit. We recovered post coronary angioplasty and stent placement patients who came directly from the cardiac catheterization lab.

I was a new charge nurse on an extremely busy night. Our hospital had two cath labs and they had procedures scheduled throughout the shift. Each RN could have up to four patients. Patty, one of the nurses, had three fresh stent patients and another on the way. She was understandably overwhelmed by this assignment, so I volunteered to take the patient coming from the cath lab, a 55 year-old male named Mr. *K*. I stated that I would take full responsibility for his care and we would re-evaluate her assignment in three hours to see if I could transfer him back to her. Patty agreed and was very relieved to focus on recovering her other patients.

Mr. *K* arrived from the cath lab in stable condition. After getting him settled and doing a complete assessment, I checked his orders. Like most post-stent patients, Mr. *K* had an order for 15 mg of Coumadin to be given *stat*.

I went to the med room to get the Coumadin. As I was walking back to his room, I passed Patty in the hallway. I had a strange feeling that she had come from Mr. *K*'s room and that she may have given Mr. *K* his Coumadin already. But instead of speaking to Patty about it, I asked Mr. *K* if he had been given any medications since coming to our unit. He said no. Since he was alert and oriented, I gave him the Coumadin. When I got back to the nurse's station, Patty said: "I gave Mr. *K* his Coumadin." My heart sank, and I ran down to his room to check on him – why I don't know – his 30 mg of Coumadin wouldn't have an effect on him for at least 24 hours.

As I walked back to the nurse's station in a panic because of the med error, I passed our flex nurse, Joan, in the hallway. The flex nurse didn't have a patient assignment of her own, but instead helped us recover patients. Joan was carrying a medicine cup. Again I had a strange feeling, but this time I stopped Joan in the hallway and asked her who the medication was for. "I thought I'd help you out and give Mr. *K* his Coumadin," she replied. It was bad enough that Mr. *K* received an extra dose of Coumadin – if I hadn't stopped Joan in the hallway, he would have received a third dose of Coumadin that night!

Patty refused to accept any responsibility for the med error – she insisted that it was entirely my fault. I notified the physician of the error and filled out an *Unusual Occurrence Report* about what happened.

I wasn't scheduled to work for a few days, but I was so worried that something would happen to Mr. *K*, that I called each shift to check on him. As it turned out, he didn't have any negative physical effects from the extra Coumadin dose, but it did add an extra day to his hospital stay.

After reviewing the incident, my supervisor concluded that the error was Patty's and not mine. I didn't agree – I think Patty and I were both responsible for this mistake.

What I learned from the incident was the vital link between clear communication and patient safety. When I told Patty I would assume Mr. *K*'s care for three hours, I should have clarified exactly what this meant. I also realized I should have followed my instincts and talked to Patty directly when I suspected she was in the patient's room. Most importantly, we discovered that our system for administering medications to patients admitted directly from the cath lab was dangerous because there was no centralized method for charting medication administration in the patient's first hour on our unit. We worked together to change the process and reduce the risk of medication errors for these patients.

Regulation of Quality Improvement in Health Care

Today quality improvement is embraced, supported and regulated on several fronts. Collaboration between health care professionals, non-profit organizations and government agencies, all committed to improving our health care system and the quality of care we provide, has led to numerous quality improvement activities. The Institute of Medicine (IOM), The Joint Commission (JC), Center for Medicare and Medicaid (CMS), Agency for Healthcare Research and Quality (AHRQ), National Quality Forum (NQF), Institute for Healthcare Improvement (IHI) and the American Nurses Association (ANA) are some of the major organizations and agencies driving quality improvement activities. In this section, we'll describe some of their most notable initiatives and recommendations.

The health care quality movement gained traction when President Clinton commissioned a special advisory committee to look at the US health care system in the 1990s. Their findings prompted the Institute of Medicine (IOM), a private, nonprofit recommending body whose work is based on research, to publish *The Quality Chasm*, a series of reports that shaped our approaches to quality improvement and patient safety. The IOM's 2001 report, *Crossing the Quality Chasm: A New Health System for the 21st Century*, defined quality as "the degree to which health services for individuals and populations increase the likelihood of desired health outcomes and are consistent with professional knowledge." Their 2003 publication, *Patient Safety: Achieving a New Standard of Care*, connected quality improvement activities to patient safety – defining patient safety as "freedom from accidental injury."

However it was the 1999 IOM report, *To Err is Human*, that recommended our country's health system focus on five key areas to ensure quality across the continuum:

- Provide leadership

- Recognize human limits in process design

- Promote effective teams

- Anticipate the unexpected

- Create a learning environment

As we mentioned earlier in this chapter, leaders have the responsibility to create the environment for quality and patient safety to thrive. They provide the vision and support for making quality the priority of all staff members. Creating the environment for quality improvement activities to thrive requires the creation of cultures of trust, respect and acceptance of human error. It requires leaders to embrace a *Just Culture*.

Because the IOM has no enforcement powers, their recommendations are generally carried out by governmental agencies, professional associations and/or coalitions, including, but not limited to:

Agency for Health Care Research and Quality (AHRQ) – Housed within the Federal Department of Health and Human Services, AHRQ's core mission is to improve the quality, safety, efficiency and effectiveness of health care for all Americans. AHRQ supports research to improve the quality of health care services and helps individuals make informed health care decisions. This agency has a history of funding and partnering with organizations and health systems to improve patient care and develop tools to sustain long-term quality improvement activities.

National Quality Forum (NQF) – A nonprofit organization originally created by health care leaders from the public and private sectors to promote and ensure patient protection and health care quality through measurement and public reporting. Today NQF's mission is to improve the quality of our American health care system. NQF developed the list of *Never Events*, a compilation of preventable adverse health events that should *never* occur in the health care setting. Examples of *Never Events* include: surgery on the wrong body part; death or serious disability associated with a fall occurring in a health care institution; and a stage 3 or 4 pressure ulcer acquired after admission to a health care facility. NQF's diverse membership includes consumer organizations, public and private purchasers, clinicians, hospitals, and accrediting and certifying agencies, as well as health care research and quality improvement organizations. They are one of the most respected and successful conveners of coalitions to drive continuous quality improvement activities.

Institute for Healthcare Improvement (IHI) – IHI is a worldwide leader and innovator in health and health care improvement. This nonprofit organization was formed in the 1980s by visionary leaders committed to creating an improved health system focused on quality and patient safety. IHI often uses the *Plan-Do-Study-Act* (PDSA) process to test potential improvements on a small scale, prior to implementing the large scale changes that ultimately transform practice and improve patient care. As we mentioned earlier, IHI partnered with the Robert Wood Johnson Foundation to create the Transforming Care at the Bedside (TCAB) project.

The Joint Commission (JC) – The JC accredits the majority of hospitals and health systems in the US, as well as many hospitals in other countries. A non-profit organization, the JC's mission is to evaluate health care organizations and motivate providers to excel at delivering safe and effective care. The JC collaborates with the Centers for Medicare and Medicaid (CMS) on *Core Measures* (more information about *Core Measures* later in this chapter), assists facilities with strategies to achieve excellence in patient care and conducts public awareness campaigns to recognize hospitals for outstanding performance.

The JC has played an active role in developing national patient safety standards by spearheading the National Patient Safety Goals (NPSG) program. Today, these safety goals are a critical method by which the JC fosters and enforces major changes in patient safety. The JC brings together interdisciplinary experts along with consumers and stakeholders to address emerging patient safety issues. The JC collaborates with this advisory group to determine high priority patient safety issues and best practice approaches to address these issues. The information is then distributed to the appropriate entities to ensure implementation. Examples of what the NPSG program has addressed include:

- Look-alike/sound-alike drugs
- "Do Not Use" abbreviations
- Communication among the health care team
- Hospital-acquired infections

RNs Take an Active Role in Quality Improvement

"The very first requirement in a hospital is that it should do no harm."

Florence Nightingale

Care redesign and restructuring swept through our nation's health systems in the early 1990s. While innovation in care delivery was embraced by nurse leaders, they soon discovered there was no data available to guide decision-making. In 1995, the ANA released its *Report Card on Nursing*. This report challenged RNs to work collaboratively to identify key nurse-sensitive indicators – nursing interventions that directly affect patient safety and quality care.

The National Database for Nursing Quality Indicators (NDNQI) and the Collaborative Alliance for Nursing Outcomes (CALNOC) are two organizations that were formed in response to ANA's challenge. Both NDNQI and CALNOC have contributed to the National Qualilty Forum's (NQF) nurse-sensitive metrics. CALNOC has been at the forefront of providing actionable information and research on nurse-sensitive indicators to participating hospitals for more than 15 years.

Your authors have had the privilege of working with the CALNOC team. Hospitals participating in the CALNOC registry have made significant improvements in quality of care, especially for patients at risk for hospital-acquired pressure ulcers (HAPUs). CALNOC's work on medication administration accuracy has been one of the most innovative nurse sensitive programs developed to date. Both CALNOC and NDNQI are testaments to the positive influence nurses have on quality and patient safety through leadership, research and direct care.

Magnet Recognition Program

Nursing excellence, innovation and quality patient care are three major hallmarks of *Magnet* facilities. To achieve *Magnet* recognition from the American Nurses Credentialing Center (ANCC), hospitals undertake a rigorous application process followed by an intense site survey. *Magnet* facilities must demonstrate excellence in nursing practice and adherence to national patient care standards. At the core of a *Magnet* hospital is an empowered professional nursing staff committed to evidence-based practice, embracing professional autonomy and supporting interdisciplinary collaboration, communication and cooperation.

Many hospitals across the nation are either *Magnet* recognized facilities, on the journey to attain *Magnet* recognition or have embraced many of the program principles known as *Forces of Magnetism*. For hospitals that don't have the resources to obtain *Magnet* recognition, ANCC created the *Pathway to Excellence*, an alternative program to recognize positive practice environments where nurses excel.

The Forces of Magnetism

The *Forces of Magnetism* are attributes or outcomes that exemplify nursing excellence and provide the framework for the *Magnet Recognition Program*. The 14 *Forces of Magnetism* are:

Quality of Nurse Leadership – Knowledgeable, strong, risk-taking nurse leaders follow a strategic and visionary philosophy, and convey a strong sense of advocacy and support for the staff and the patient.

Organizational Structure – Dynamic and responsive to change; decentralized decision-making prevails with strong nursing representation.

Management Style – The health care organization and nursing leaders create an environment supporting participation by being visible, accessible and committed to effective communication.

Personnel Policies and Programs – Creative and flexible staffing models support a safe and healthy work environment.

Quality of Care – Quality is the systematic driving force for nursing and the organization, positively influencing patient outcomes.

Quality Improvement – Structures are in place for the measurement of quality and programs for improving quality of care and services.

Consultation and Resources – Adequate resources, support and opportunities are provided. The organization promotes involvement of nurses in professional organizations and community projects.

Autonomy – The RN assesses and provides appropriate nursing actions based on competence, professional expertise and knowledge.

Community and Health Care Organization – Strong partnerships support improved client outcomes and the health of communities.

Nurses as Teachers – Professional nurses are involved in educational activities within the organization and community. Students from a variety of academic programs are welcomed and supported.

Image of Nursing – Nurses are viewed as integral to the health care organization's ability to provide patient care.

Interdisciplinary Relationships – Collaborative working relationships among the disciplines are encouraged and valued.

Professional Development – The health care organization values and supports the personal and professional growth and development of staff.

Retrieved from: www.nursecredentialing.org/magnet/programoverview/history magnetprograms

Health Care Reform

The *Patient Protection and Affordable Care Act* (ACA) is the most significant health care legislation since Medicare was enacted in 1965. The goal of this 906-page comprehensive piece of legislation is to decrease cost, increase access and improve care. The ACA expands health care coverage to 32 million people through a combination of public and private sector insurance expansions and reform of the system.

Someone once said that the Affordable Care Act provides a road map for health care reform – the only problem is that there is no road! Now is the time to create the new road to improve health care services for our patients and communities.

The ACA is full of opportunities for collaboration, standardization, innovation, coordination and dissemination of quality improvement initiatives. Nurses play an active role in the implementation of health care reform. Our profession has the opportunity to make a significant impact in the areas of patient outcomes, coordination of care and decreasing health care costs. As we develop innovative models of care, new roles for nurses will emerge.

Value-Based Purchasing

Hospital Value-Based Purchasing (HVBP) was established by the ACA to hold health care providers accountable for quality and cost of care. This initiative gives financial incentives to hospitals based on the quality of care they provide to Medicare and Medicaid patients. As part of this program, the Centers for Medicare and Medicaid (CMS) are reducing base payments to hospitals. These reductions are expected to increase over the next several years. The withheld funds will then be used as incentive payments for hospitals based on their quality scores.

Major elements of HVBP:

• Measure and report comparative performance data for hospitals.
• Reimburse providers based on quality and performance.
• Offer incentives to encourage individuals to select high value services and better manage their health.

CMS has developed a weighted system for this incentive reimbursement process. Patients' care experience and clinical processes of care will be the first domains used to measure performance improvement under this program. This new incentive process is based on continuous improvement. Therefore, the status quo is not an option if facilities want to receive incentive reimbursement. CMS is a leader in incentivizing facilities to improve quality. Other payers often follow CMS mandates and are embracing HVBP.

"No matter where your career takes you, always strive to provide quality, compassionate care."

Karen Price-Gharzeddine

Read Karen's story, *Easing a Patient's Difficult Journey*, on page 200.

Patients' Care Experience (HCAHPS)

Years before the ACA was signed into law, CMS and AHRQ began measuring hospitalized patients' perceptions of care. The Hospital Consumer Assessment of Healthcare Providers and Systems (HCAHPS) survey was developed to achieve three major goals. First, the development of a standardized survey to provide meaningful information for the consumer that's comparable for similar hospital types. The second objective was to create incentives for hospitals to improve care. The final goal was to increase accountability of hospitals for the care they provide by publicly reporting survey results.

Those involved in this work adopted rigorous multi-phase processes to ensure the validity and reliability of HCAHPS. Today HCAHPS scores are tied to hospital reimbursement. Although the scoring process is complex, the bottom line is that better scores or a hospital's continued improvement over time equates to higher incentivized reimbursement.

As HVBP is implemented, it is expected that 30 percent of reimbursement will be determined by HCAHPS scores. This percentage is expected to remain constant in recognition of the importance of the patient care experience.

As nurses we have a tremendous impact on HCAHPS scores and, as a result, our hospital's reimbursement. We will discuss how nurses can positively impact HCAHPS scores later in this chapter.

Clinical Processes of Care (Core Measures)

Core Measures = the right patient, right care at the right time!

Core Measures are evidence-based standards of care that have been shown to improve clinical outcomes. Hospitals are required to report *Core Measures* to both CMS and the Joint Commission. Since 2004, CMS and the JC have been working to align measures to streamline the process and avoid duplication.

Core Measure scores in the clinical areas of acute myocardial infarction, heart failure, pneumonia, surgical care improvements and healthcare-associated infections will be used to compute reimbursement for the clinical processes of care domain in the HVBP program (see box on next page for an example of *Core Measures*). The HVBP benchmark for many of the required indicators is 100 percent, making it necessary to get these *Core Measures* right every time to ensure optimal incentivized reimbursement.

It is expected that other metrics will be added to the HVBP program over the next few years. Hospital-acquired conditions, mortality index and patient safety indicators will likely be included in the next phase of the program. Because CMS encourages cost effective care, an efficiency measure may also be added.

Sample Core Measure Set

Acute Myocardial Infarction

- Aspirin on arrival
- Aspirin prescribed at discharge
- Angiotensin converting enzyme inhibitor or angiotensin receptor blocker prescribed for left ventricular systolic dysfunction
- Adult smoking cessation advice/counseling offered
- Beta-blocker prescribed at discharge
- Fibrinolytic therapy received within 30 minutes of hospital arrival
- Median time to primary percutaneous coronary intervention *(within 90 minutes of hospital arrival in centers providing these services)*
- Statin prescribed at discharge

If any of these interventions are contra-indicated for a specific patient, this must be noted in the documentation.

Consumers, the government and third-party payers want quality. If consumers don't perceive they've received quality care, they can impact a hospital's bottom line by giving low marks on HCAPHS or seeking care elsewhere. Regulators can cite and fine facilities for providing poor care and third party payers can cancel contracts. Acute care facilities are no longer going to be reimbursed for hospital-acquired conditions or re-admissions within a specified window of time.

The care you provide as a member of the health care team directly affects the safety and well-being of your patients as well as the reimbursement your hospital receives.

"...behind all of the machines, noise, lines and chaos of the NICU, there is a child, a human being whose life depends on the care I give." Heaven Holdbrooks

Read Heaven's story, *The Best, Worst Experience*, on page 210.

Quality is About What You Bring to the Clinical Environment

"Evidence-based practice is the integration of best clinical practice, research evidence, nursing expertise, and the values and preferences of the individuals, families and communities who are served."

Sigma Theta Tau International

Now let's turn our attention to what you bring to the nursing team as a new graduate. In the area of quality improvement you have a great deal to offer. You have been exposed to evidence-based practice and its application in the clinical arena as well as the IOM's quality competencies for professionals. Technology has also been a tool that you've mastered as part of your academic preparation. As a result, you may have skills and knowledge that other members of the team may not yet possess.

In 2003, the IOM released the report, *Health Professions Education: A Bridge to Quality*, which clearly identified a gap between education and practice. The report suggested that health care education failed to keep pace with the ever-changing health care quality movement. This report identified five core competencies that needed to be integrated into the academic programs for all health care disciplines to ensure that quality and patient safety is a priority in the training of health care professionals. Nursing modified the competencies slightly by separating quality from safety. The core competencies in nursing curriculum include:

- Patient-centered care
- Teamwork and collaboration – interprofessionally-focused
- Evidence-based practice
- Quality improvement
- Safety
- Informatics

Building on these core competencies, academic leaders began the Quality and Safety Education for Nurses (QSEN) project, with funding from the Robert Wood Johnson Foundation. The purpose of this three-phase project was to prepare our future nurses with the knowledge, skills and attitudes (KSAs) necessary to practice in environments where continuous quality improvement thrives. Nursing programs across the country have embraced QSEN as the standard for quality improvement education.

As a new graduate, you're the first generation whose curriculum included the IOM's core professional competencies. Your colleagues and peers, who were educated prior to the adoption of QSEN in nursing school programs, may not be familiar with the IOM core competencies or QSEN. As a result, your potential contributions to the quality improvement activities on your unit can be significant.

As nursing students, you were exposed to the latest research and evidence as well as strategies for integrating evidence into practice. More importantly, you have the knowledge and skills to access information using technology. As questions or issues surface, you can offer your expertise in bringing information and data to the team as they strive for better ways of providing care. The challenge will be how you, as a new staff member and recent graduate, make those contributions in a positive way so that your message is heard. Once again, effective communication skills are a key factor in your nursing role – this time to improve patient care and outcomes.

Today's technology allows us to access new research and evidence immediately. The Cochrane Collaborative Library (www.cochrane.org) or the Joanna Briggs Institute (JBI) (www.joannabriggs.edu.au) are two examples of sites providing systematic reviews and EBP guidelines to help clinicians transfer research into practice. The JBI program actually has a software system that helps clinicians judge if the study or studies being reviewed actually support identified interventions. Your employer may subscribe to one of these important resources. If so, be sure to take advantage of these tools.

Quality is About What You Give

When we asked veteran nurse leaders what they believed is the most important message for new RNs related to quality improvement, their responses were similar: "treat every patient the way you would want your loved ones treated."

What a powerful concept! Always strive to provide your patients with the same level of care you would want given to members of your family. Be open to new and better ways of providing care. Look for evidence to drive change if the current modalities aren't good enough. Advocate for change when the research identifies better methods. Let your work be driven by evidence and passion so that you provide the best possible care to every patient, every time – because that's exactly what you would want for your loved ones.

"Treat every patient the way you would want your loved ones treated!" Stephanie Mearns

Your Impact on the Patient Experience Domain

Each and every day on your patient care unit, you can influence your patients' perception of care. When we treat patients with respect, compassion and approach each patient encounter as an educational opportunity, patients receive optimal care, and their perceptions of the care experience are usually very positive.

You'll have the satisfaction of providing the best care possible, and your actions can also impact your hospital's financial viability. Remember, a hospital's reimbursement is tied to the eight value-based measures found in the HCAHPS survey. Here are some specific ways you can positively influence your patients' perception of their care:

Communication with the Nurse – Hospitalization is a frightening time for patients and families. As we discussed in Chapter 4, people often don't absorb information or communicate effectively during periods of stress and anxiety. As the RN, you can often ease your patient's anxiety and, as a result, increase their openness to learning about their condition and treatment.

When you initially meet your patient, introduce yourself as the RN in charge of their care for that particular shift. Let them know how long you'll be working with them and how to reach you if they need immediate assistance. Take time to ask about their primary concerns related to their hospitalization. Listen to what they're saying so that together you can develop a plan to address these concerns. Share critical details about the patient with appropriate members of the interdisciplinary team, so that together the team can provide the best care possible. Always pass on information about the patient's priorities and their perception of care to the oncoming shift.

Communication with the Doctor – While we don't have control over the interactions our patients have with their physicians, we can help our patients understand the medical plan of care. Joint rounds by the MD and RN minimize confusion over orders and allows the nurse to fully explain the interdisciplinary plan of care as needed. Joint rounds also provide an opportunity for you as the RN to advocate for your patients, especially if they don't share their questions or concerns about their care with the MD. Some patients, particularly the elderly, are hesitant to ask questions or raise concerns because they perceive that it's disrespectful of the MD's authority. As an RN, it is your professional responsibility to be an advocate for your patients.

Responsiveness of Hospital Staff – Patients are often anxious, afraid or require assistance with activities of daily living. When they push their call lights, they expect staff to respond in a timely manner. When discussing the plan of care with your patient, include information about pain management and toileting routines. Reassure your patient that you'll be rounding hourly to check on their pain, toileting needs and any other requests. Taking a few minutes at the start of the shift to discuss patient needs will save you and your colleagues time later. When you focus on patients' needs and questions up front, they feel included and their anxiety usually decreases.

Pain Management – Effective pain management is more than just administering medications. Pain is very personal and subjective. Comfort measures such as a cool compress, a soothing back rub, repositioning, and speaking in a calm, reassuring voice can help reduce anxiety and alleviate pain. Ask your patients what works for them – they will help determine an appropriate treatment plan.

Cleanliness and Quietness of the Hospital Environment – As nurses, we're responsible for ensuring that our patients' rooms are safe and free of clutter. Incorporating the "backward glance" as part of your routine will help remind you to look back before leaving a patient's room to ensure it's free from clutter and there are no visible hazards.

Also ensure that their environment is conducive to rest and healing by minimizing noise. Use a quiet voice and urge your colleagues to do the same, especially on the night shift.

Communication About Medicines – The HCAHPS survey asks questions related to patients' understanding of the medications they received. Approach each medication pass as an opportunity to educate your patients about their meds, including why they're receiving them, the medication's basic actions and potential side effects.

Discharge Planning – Preparing a patient for discharge from the hospital should begin on admission. Inquire about your patient's plans for discharge. The earlier you identify needs, the easier it will be to put systems in place for a safe handoff to the next level of care or the transition home.

Overall Rating of Hospital – Patients will be asked to provide an overall rating for the hospital stay. If their personal needs haven't been satisfied, then the overall rating of the hospital will suffer.

"Great care happens when one human being truly connects with another." Donna Kistler

Read Donna's story, *Making the Human Connection*, on page 202.

As professionals and employees, we want to work at great facilities. Should you need care, where do you want to be treated? If you didn't list your current hospital, then why would patients? Ask yourself: What can I do to make this hospital stay more comfortable for my patient? How can I meet my patient's needs? The answers to these questions will guide you in removing barriers to quality patient care.

In Conclusion - Putting It All Together

Quality and patient safety initiatives can be complex and change rapidly. What do you need to know as a newly licensed nurse?

• Patient safety is your number one priority.

• As a professional, it's your responsibility to be part of the quality improvement process. RNs have a direct impact on quality care and patient safety. You possess the knowledge, but not the experience, to determine when improvements are needed. By partnering with your preceptor and RN colleagues – you can have a positive impact on the quality of patient care.

• Recognize your responsibility and authority in the implementation of processes associated with improvements in patient safety and quality.

• Learn what your unit indicators are and the metrics associated with these measures. The status quo isn't good enough – we must continue to improve the care we provide to patients.

• Use your voice when you see deviations from the standards that may result in potential or actual harm, and/or when you have evidence supporting change.

• Strive to improve your communication skills. When we effectively communicate with our patients, their families and members of the interdisciplinary team, we have the potential to improve the quality of care patients receive. Review Chapters 4 and 5 in this book, utilize the tools in our reference list and attend classes to help you build your communication skills.

• Don't assume – ask questions and seek clarity! When we make assumptions, quality and patient safety are often put at risk.

• If you're unsure about something, then ask – your questions may bring up ideas or thoughts that could have a direct impact on the quality of care.

• Recognize distractions – know yourself. Identify the distractions interfering with your ability to provide excellence in patient care.

- Focus on the task at hand.

- If you are stressed, stop and re-evaluate – know your personal triggers and take a timeout before you get to the point where you may make an error.

Knowing Your Triggers

Pat shares this story:

Reading can be a challenge for me. Over the years, I've learned that my reading difficulty intensifies when I'm stressed. Written numbers and words begin to appear mixed and out of order. After making a medication error because I transposed the dosages of two different medications, I realized I needed to take a timeout when I found myself in situations where I felt overwhelmed and stressed.

While I was truly thankful that my patient wasn't harmed by my error, I accepted both the personal and professional accountability for the error without making excuses. My error was not a system error, knowledge deficit or skill deficit – it was a human error.

My medication error taught me never to administer medications when I was feeling overwhelmed and stressed, and to take a "timeout" if necessary. If a timeout wasn't an option, I would ask a colleague to verify the medication and dosage with me. I adopted several other safeguards to ensure patient safety.

As a new graduate, I encourage you to recognize your personal trigger points and take a timeout or utilize other strategies so that your stress doesn't cause you to make an error. If you do make an error, use it as a learning experience to improve your practice.

Make Quality and Patient Safety Your Priority

Quality is a team sport! Every member of the health care team must make patient safety and quality care their number one priority. Seems pretty simple – *right?* So why are patients still dying from medical errors? Why do we need the government to include performance improvement as part of the *Affordable Care Act?* Why? Because we're humans who work in highly complex, hectic and, at times, chaotic environments. This isn't an excuse – it's a fact!

As RNs we not only have a professional responsibility, but we're positioned to be active participants in the quest to improve patient care. The opportunities for nurses to make significant advances in the quality of care we provide to patients and communities are endless!

Questions for Reflection

1. Ask your preceptor or manager to share your facility's HCAHPS scores. Are there areas for improvement? Select one or two areas for improvement from the patient experience scores. What actions will you implement to help to improve these scores?

2. You're working on the day shift. In reviewing your patient's chart you noticed that the patient didn't receive their 6 a.m. dose of an anti-hypertensive. It's now 10 a.m. What actions would you take in reporting this situation? Who should be involved in the investigation? Do you consider this error in omission a medication error? Does your facility consider this an adverse event? Why?

3. You must perform a wound irrigation and sterile dressing change for one of your patients. You asked another RN to assist you. You wash your hands prior to the procedure but notice that the other RN does not. How should you handle this situation?

4. You've been reading about a new care delivery model that's grounded in research. The evidence indicates that patient outcomes are improved by this model. Discuss strategies for introducing this new practice on your unit.

Endless Possibilities: Looking Beyond Your 1st Job

"If there is one thing I could inject in every young nurse, it would be the notion that you should approach possibilities with a 'why not' attitude, rather than finding a million reasons for not going forward." Marla Salmon, ScD, RN, FAAN

Nursing is a career of infinite possibilities! When you begin your first job as a nurse, you're focused on transitioning to your new role as an RN. Later as you move through the stages of novice to expert and feel more comfortable and confident in your RN role, you'll begin to think about the next steps in your career.

In this chapter, we'll provide strategies to help you take charge of you career path so that you can enjoy a long and prosperous journey as a registered nurse.

Embrace Lifelong Learning

Throughout this book, we've talked about the benefits of lifelong learning. Commitment to lifelong learning is one of the hallmarks of a professional. As you move forward in your career, we strongly encourage you to return to school to pursue another degree. Maybe you have an associate degree in nursing. Consider obtaining a bachelor's degree. Already have a BSN? Then think about a master's or doctorate degree.

In 2010, the Institute of Medicine (IOM), in partnership with the Robert Wood Johnson Foundation, released the groundbreaking report, *The Future of Nursing: Leading Change, Advancing Health*. The report provides a framework for nurses to transform our profession and improve the health of patients and communities. Of the report's eight key recommendations, three focus on education and lifelong learning. The IOM report recommends that by the year 2020, 80 percent of nurses should be educated at the baccalaureate level and the number of RNs with doctorate degrees should double from 2010 levels.

The third recommendation related to education promotes lifelong learning more generally, stating that RNs should "continue their education and engage in lifelong learning to gain the competencies needed to provide care for diverse populations across the lifespan."

Advancing your nursing education will further enhance your development as a professional nurse and enable you to provide optimal care for your patients. It will also open doors to a myriad of opportunities in nursing. Right now you're focused on transitioning from new graduate to professional nurse. As your career progresses and you feel more comfortable and confident in your role as an RN, consider returning to school. Whenever possible, attend continuing education courses, grand rounds and other opportunities to expand your knowledge and skills.

Building Your Professional Toolkit Through Additional Education

Pat shares this story:

I had been working as a relief charge nurse in the ICU when our hospital's chief nursing officer asked me to try a new role she was developing on the neurosurgical unit. I felt honored that she selected me to help her and the unit manager develop this role, which closely resembled a clinical nurse specialist. In this position, I would serve as a unit educator and a conduit between the neurosurgeons and nursing staff to aid in the management of complex neuro patients.

I embraced this new role with enthusiasm and a sense of professional pride. The staff was most welcoming and the unit manager and I had worked together previously. I was even given the opportunity to enhance my skills by attending an eight-week program in neurosurgical nursing. By all measures this seemed to be a career move made in heaven.

I loved working one-on-one with the nursing staff and enjoyed collaborating with the physicians, especially assisting with diagnostic procedures. But other aspects of the role were very difficult. I soon realized I didn't possess the skills or academic preparation to be successful. While I was a great clinician, I didn't know the first thing about program or curriculum development.

With my head held high, I went to see the CNO. I explained that while I valued the opportunity to try something new, I regrettably didn't have the appropriate skill set to make a difference for the nursing staff or patients.

I could have gone back to the ICU and continued my career, but instead I took this opportunity to evaluate my long-term goals. I decided I wanted to achieve the goal of becoming a clinical nurse specialist. But as an associate degree graduate, I knew I needed more education to accomplish my objective – so I enrolled in school.

I eventually became a clinical nurse specialist at this same hospital. This time, I had the academic preparation and professional tools to make a difference for the staff and patients, and create a more rewarding career experience for myself.

Obtaining Certification in Your Specialty Area

Certification signifies expertise, clinical judgment and achievement in a specific area of nursing. It's the formal process in which a certifying organization validates a nurse's knowledge, skills and abilities in a practice area, such as critical care, oncology, case management, etc. Nurses achieve certification through education, experience and passage of a qualifying exam in the specific clinical area.

The American Nurses Credentialing Center offers a variety of certifications. In addition, many specialty organizations, including the American Association of Critical Care Nurses, Oncology Nursing Society, Emergency Nurses Association and American Association of Women's Health, Obstetric and Neonatal Nurses, offer certifications in their specific area of clinical practice.

Obtaining certification in your clinical area enhances your nursing practice, clinical expertise and credibility as a professional. Most employers recognize that certification signifies dedication and commitment. As a result, certification in a specialty area will often give you the edge when pursuing career advancement opportunities. To learn more about the requirements and process for certification in your specialty, visit your specialty organization's national website.

Find a Mentor

Although we thoroughly covered the subject of mentors in Chapter 2 (*Paving the Road: Preceptors, Mentors and Role Models*), the importance of mentors to your career success bears repeating. A mentor is someone who will help you grow personally and professionally through advice, guidance and providing a safe, non-threatening environment to discuss ideas. Mentors will often recognize qualities you may not see in yourself. They help you develop these talents and abilities and reach your full potential.

As you progress in your career, please make the commitment to share your knowledge and expertise by precepting and mentoring others. Always remember what it's like to be a novice. Help other RNs, just as other colleagues have helped you. This is one of the most important ways we can give back to our profession and help new nurses achieve success. In addition, you'll find these relationships extremely rewarding.

Join Professional Organizations

As we discussed in Chapter 3 (*Defining Your Role as an RN: Important Resources to Guide Your Practice*), supporting our profession by belonging to one or more nursing organizations is one of the hallmarks of a professional. The American Nurses Association is the organization for all RNs. There are also numerous specialty organizations for your areas of interest or expertise in nursing.

Professional organizations provide information and resources to help you excel in your practice. By becoming involved in these organizations, you can take advantage of networking opportunities to build important professional contacts and meet potential mentors. Through networking and collaboration with members of your professional organization, you'll have opportunities to influence practice, participate in research and continue to grow professionally. Professional organizations, such as ANA and Oncology Nursing Society, welcome new graduates and offer newly licensed RNs discounts on membership.

Look for Opportunities within Your Department

There are opportunities within your nursing department to expand your skills and build your expertise. These may include: serving on a committee, assisting with quality projects, gathering data, drafting policies, providing inservice training and precepting students and new staff members. As a recent graduate, your expertise with technology can be extremely helpful in departments where staff may be struggling with the electronic medical record and other recent technological advances.

Expanding your skills beyond patient care helps you build your professional toolkit and exposes you to other aspects of nursing you may find rewarding. Speak to your manager about potential projects within your nursing department.

Looking for Opportunities to Expand Your Skills

Brenda shares this story:

I was an RN for five years when I started thinking about moving from acute care to another area of nursing. I always enjoyed teaching and precepting new employees and students, so I began to explore whether a position as a nurse educator would be right for me.

When I met with my manager for my annual performance appraisal, she asked what my long-term career goals were. I mentioned my love of teaching, but relayed my apprehension that I wasn't sure I'd enjoy doing it full time. She replied: "If you want more exposure to teaching, I can certainly help you with that."

She opened her desk drawer and handed me two *Unusual Occurrence Reports,* saying: "In the last month, we've had two errors related to blood administration. Would you do a 20-minute refresher on this topic at our next staff meeting?" I presented the blood administration inservice and received good feedback from my colleagues. I began working on other education-related projects for the manager, and eventually 16 hours per month of my time became allocated to departmental education programs.

We formed an education committee and I was appointed chair. Several RNs were interested in serving on the committee and providing more educational opportunities for our health care team. We revamped our orientation process, provided training for preceptors, convinced some of our cardiologists to deliver lectures for staff and utilized the expertise of more experienced RNs to present both formal classes for newer nurses and short educational offerings during staff meetings.

Not only did these endeavors enhance the nursing practice on our unit, they also gave me the opportunity to build my program planning and presentation skills. These early experiences were a great asset when I later transferred to an educator position in the hospital's staff development department.

Charting Your Path: Be Open to Possibilities

If you're considering changing jobs or looking for other opportunities in nursing, we encourage you to explore the wide variety of career paths in our profession. Many nurses, especially newer ones, aren't aware of the many avenues they can pursue in nursing. The first step in this process is taking a personal inventory.

Questions to Consider for Your Personal Inventory

- What are my interests and passions in nursing?
- What aspects of my current job do I enjoy most?
- Are there things I wish I could do in my current job, or would like to do more of?
- What are my strengths?
- What am I best at?
- What skills/abilities would I like to develop?

After you've identified your passions and strengths, consider what nursing roles fit your interests and abilities. Talk to more experienced nurses to gain insights. Explore various roles within and outside your organization. Then determine if this is a role you can move into with your current qualifications or if additional education, training and/or experience is necessary. Perhaps you're interested in moving from your med/surg unit to the emergency department. Obtaining *Advanced Cardiac Life Support* (ACLS) and *Pediatric Advanced Life Support* (PALS) certifications may be required before applying for a position in the ED. Or maybe you want to move from acute care to public health nursing. Do you have a BSN? Do you have a public health nursing certificate? Learning about the requirements of the roles you're interested in will help you successfully plot your career path.

Learning More About Other Nursing Roles

If you're considering a job change to a different area, but are hesitant because you're not sure you'll really like it, you have some options:

- Talk to nurses already in the role – you can gain valuable insights about the role and what qualifications are needed.

- Job shadowing – contact the department manager and tell them you're interested in possibly pursuing a job in their area. They will often be open to allowing you to shadow a nurse in the department, especially if you're employed in the organization.

"I learned the importance of being open to new possibilities and being accepting of opportunities that come your way – even if it's not what you anticipated." Carrie Garland

Read Carries's story, *Forging New Paths*, on page 266.

• Interim roles – there may be an interim job in the department that you can fill in order to see if you're suited for the position. This is especially prevalent if you're considering changing roles within your organization. Perhaps your current manager will allow you to temporarily reduce your hours in your home department, so that you can work some shifts in the department you're interested in.

For example: Tom is an RN in the surgical ICU. He's interested in working in his hospital's quality department. One of the RNs in the department will be out for four weeks on medical leave. The quality department manager and Tom's manager are willing to let him work in the quality department two days per week for the next four weeks. During that time, Tom will reduce his ICU schedule to two days a week.

This isn't an unusual practice, especially if you have a supportive manager. You'll never know unless you ask.

Trying Out the Job Through an Interim Role

Brenda shares this story:

I was a nurse educator in a staff development department that was part of a large hospital system. One of our sister hospitals was in a rural area about 15 miles outside the region our education department served.

One day, my manager told me the rural hospital needed an interim education manager for 2-3 months until they could hire a permanent one. I had previously expressed an interest in management and we had discussed strategies for me to make that career move. The problem was, I wasn't sure if management was a direction I wanted to pursue. This interim management opportunity seemed like a perfect way to test the role. So I accepted the position.

I loved the job, the hospital and the education team! After three months, I assumed the position on a permanent basis and stayed in the role for three years. It was one of the best jobs I've had in my nursing career. I never would have applied for the permanent position without first having the opportunity to try it out on an interim basis. I was very thankful I had such a supportive manager to help me explore career options.

"Once you discover your interests in the many fields you can pursue as an RN, expose yourself to that role as much as possible and network with colleagues in that specialty area. In the end, it will open doors for many opportunities to come." Veanne O'Neill

Read Veanne's story, *Designing Your Road Map for Success*, on page 272.

Finding Your Niche: What if Your Current Job Isn't Working Out?

Nursing is a profession with many career paths. If you're in a job that doesn't feel rewarding or worthwhile, this doesn't necessarily mean that nursing isn't the right career for you. Unfortunately, of the new nurses who leave our profession, many do so because their first job doesn't work out for them.

If your job isn't right for you – don't leave the profession, leave the job! But before you make a move, analyze why you're unhappy in your present position. Possibilities to consider:

• **Work environment** – Are your team members and/or manager not supporting you? If the team members on a particular shift aren't supporting you, discuss this with your manager. You may be able to move to a different shift within the department. If your manager isn't supportive, consider transferring to another department within the hospital, or look for another employer.

• **Your level of competence** – Do you feel that your level of competence isn't where it should be to care for the patient population on your unit? Remember the novice to expert stages of development we discussed in Chapter 1. Initially, you'll feel uncomfortable in your new role as an RN. This feeling should decrease as you gain experience. But if you believe that your comfort level and/or competence should be greater than it currently is, discuss your concerns with your manager. Perhaps you need additional time with a preceptor or could attend some continuing education classes to increase your knowledge, skills and confidence.

• **Shift/hours** – Are you working a shift that doesn't fit with your body clock or lifestyle? For example, are you working the night shift and having difficulty sleeping during the day? Is this causing you to become rundown and irritable? A change to another shift may be what's needed.

• **Clinical area of practice** – Is the patient population or type of

"Nursing is full of opportunities. Just work hard and keep seeking." Jeremy Weed

Read Jeremy's story, *Taking Control of Your Career*, on page 270.

nursing not rewarding for you? Maybe acute care isn't right for you and you'd be happier working in a clinic or outpatient setting. Or, you want to be a pediatric nurse, but took a job in acute rehab because that was the only position available. Once you get some experience under your belt, you'll have a much better chance of landing a position in your area of interest.

• **Values** – Does the organization's values clash with your personal beliefs? If so, you will probably be happier if you move to an organization that shares your values. When applying for nursing positions in other health care organizations, visit their websites to get a feel for the organization. If possible, talk to people who work there. When interviewing for positions, ask questions about the values of the organization and examples of how these values are actualized in day-to-day operations.

• **Other factors** – What other factors might be causing your displeasure with the job? Is there anything you can do to mitigate these factors in your present job, or is a change needed?

Once you analyze why you're unhappy, you'll be much better equipped to develop strategies to rectify the situation. Remember how hard you worked to become an RN. We encourage you to thoroughly examine your options before making a decision to leave the profession. If you look for your niche in nursing, there's an excellent chance you'll find it.

Taking Care of Yourself

"We need to put ourselves higher on our own 'To Do' lists!"
Michelle Obama

You can't enjoy a prosperous, fulfilling career if you're tired, stressed and living an unhealthy lifestyle. Taking care of yourself must be just as high a priority as taking care of your patients.

Compassion Fatigue

Compassion fatigue is a combination of physical, emotional and spiritual depletion associated with caring for patients and families experiencing devastating illness and traumatic episodes in their lives.

This phenomenon is not unique to nursing. Health care professionals who are repeatedly exposed to human trauma and suffering are also at risk. Other factors that can contribute to compassion fatigue are unhealthy work environments and lack of safe venues for sharing feelings associated with difficult or traumatic patient care experiences. Nurses suffering from compassion fatigue report a gradual lessening of compassion over time. This is often followed by feeling hopeless, stressed, anxious, angry and/or irritable. Other symptoms are sleeplessness and a pervasive negative attitude.

Our desire to make a difference is why many of us became RNs. Patients and families draw their strength from us during some of the most difficult times in their lives. As nurses, we're driven by a strong desire to alleviate their pain and suffering. This act of caring requires us to give of ourselves, and at times place the patient's needs before our own. However, if we don't learn to set limits and recognize the warning signs within ourselves, we will be at risk for developing compassion fatigue.

As a profession, nursing must address compassion fatigue, not only to help our colleagues, but to ensure patient safety. We know that nurses experiencing even the early onset of compassion fatigue are more likely to make mistakes or unsafe decisions, which can potentially place patients at risk. Our professional code of ethics requires us to care for ourselves, so we can competently care for others. Therefore, it's our professional obligation to seek help when we find ourselves demonstrating any of the symptoms of compassion fatigue.

The best defense against compassion fatigue is work/life balance. As a newly licensed RN there are several steps you can take to prevent compassion fatigue:

• Find a trusted preceptor, mentor or senior colleague to talk about your feelings and experiences.

• Learn to say *No!* Working extra shifts or excessive overtime depletes your energy and negatively affects your health and personal life. It's up to you to protect yourself (and your patients) when you're too tired to work an extra shift.

• Eat healthy foods and exercise regularly.

• Get enough sleep, especially if you work variable shifts.

• Nurture both professional and personal relationships.

• Discover ways to recharge your passion for nursing by attending conferences or returning to school.

• Take time off from work to rediscover other passions in your life.

Working More Than One Job

One of the wonderful attributes of our profession is the flexibility of working part-time in a variety of nursing roles. For example, Katie is an RN specializing in obstetric nursing. Katie works two shifts per week in the labor and delivery unit, one day a week in a pre-natal clinic and teaches childbirth and lactation classes 2-3 evenings per month. This combination of jobs provides Katie with three settings to pursue her passion in nursing. Her work with patients and clients in these three areas helps strengthen her nursing practice, and she thoroughly enjoys the variety.

Although this flexibility provides great opportunities to build a fulfilling career, it can be easy to over-commit. If you have multiple jobs, take care not to jeopardize your health and well-being by working too many hours per week. You also need time for family, friends and leisure activities. Don't let working too many hours rob you of this valuable time.

Because of 12-hour shifts, there are too many nurses who work two full time jobs – that's 72 hours per week! While we recognize that working two full time jobs is very lucrative financially, we believe the potential negative consequences far outweigh the financial rewards. Nurses working too many hours are prime candidates for compassion fatigue and are much more likely to make errors.

Don't put yourself, your license or your patients at risk! If you have multiple jobs, they should be part-time and allow for you to get enough rest and enjoy leisure activities.

Attaining Work/Life Balance

As we discussed in the previous section, compassion fatigue is a very real concern for health care professionals, especially nurses. Successfully balancing your personal and professional life can help you avoid compassion fatigue.

The first step is to gather data about how you spend your time. Using the grid on the following page as a guide, keep track for one week of how much time you spend in the following areas: at work, with family, with friends, pursuing hobbies, exercising, enjoying leisure activities and sleeping.

Activity	Day 1	Day 2	Day 3	Day 4	Day 5	Day 6	Day 7
Work							
Family							
Friends							
Hobbies							
Exercise							
Leisure							
Sleeping							

After collecting this data, determine the percentage of your time that you spent in each activity. Are you happy with the ways you're spending your time? For example, if you sleep eight hours per day, then 33.4 percent of your time is devoted to sleeping. How about the rest of your time? If you spend 40 percent of your time at work because you've been picking up extra shifts, how does that affect the remaining areas in your life? Are you spending enough time with your family and friends? Do you have time to exercise? What about your hobbies and leisure activities?

When we get busy with our careers, our personal lives often suffer. Maybe you squeeze a little extra time out of each day by only sleeping 5-6 hours. This may help you in the short-term, but if you continue this habit you'll jeopardize your health and increase your risk for compassion fatigue.

As an RN, you help your patients take control of their lives and health. It's up to you to do the same for your own health and well-being. By learning to pace yourself, you'll be much happier over the span of your career. Remember, your nursing career is a marathon – not the 100-yard dash!

"I encourage you to live life to its fullest and make the greatest impact you can. You will find personal satisfaction and develop into a fulfilled professional..."
Susan Herman

Read Susan's story, *Nursing: It's My Calling,* on page 258.

Questions for Reflection

1. What resources does your organization offer to promote lifelong learning? Is there an education/staff development department? Do they offer classes you're interested in? Do you have paid continuing education hours as a benefit? Tuition reimbursement? How can you use these benefits to increase your knowledge and skills and prepare for future career opportunities?

2. What are the symptoms of compassion fatigue? What personal strategies can you utilize to prevent compassion fatigue?

3. Utilizing the table on page 168, track how you spend your time for one week. How are you spending the majority of your time? Are you satisfied with the results? Are there areas you'd like to devote more time to? What changes can you make in order to bring your life into balance?

4. Your unit is under-staffed. As a result, you and your team members are often asked to work overtime and take on extra shifts. You've tried to help out by working more, but this has decreased the time you spend with your family and you haven't been able to work out at the gym as often as you'd like. You're feeling increasingly tired and irritable. There's a message on your voicemail asking you to work another extra shift tomorrow. You feel like you're letting the team down, but you just don't want to work another day this week. You must call your manager back and give her an answer. Practice strategies for tactfully saying no. What if your manager tries to persuade you to change your mind? How can you stay resolved and continue to say no?

Celebrating Nursing!

Stories of joy, passion and triumph
from RNs who travelled before you...

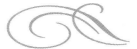

"Nursing encompasses an art, a humanistic orientation, a
feeling for the value of the individual, an intuitive sense of
ethics, and of the appropriateness of action taken."

Myrtle Aydelotte

The Essence of Nursing

My first job as a new grad was on the evening shift of a 30-bed medical/surgical/oncology unit. I learned early in my career that the true essence of nursing is the art and science of our profession blended into daily practice.

I remember vividly an experience I had during that first year, while caring for Leslie, a young male patient with leukemia. Our hospital was hundreds of miles from his home and family. I took care of Leslie for about two months and involved him in his plan of care from day one. I remember how much Leslie trusted me, and I know I made a difference in the final days of his life. His memory has never faded, and to this day stays within my heart.

I am so proud to serve as a registered nurse and nurse leader because I know we make a difference for our patients and communities every day.

Take time to journal so you never forget our meaningful work and the difference we make in the lives of our patients and their families. My early encounters with patients have guided my nursing practice and vision throughout my career and continue to influence me today.

Margarita Baggett, MSN, RN
2014 ACNL President
Graduated 1978

As a newly licensed nurse, YOU are standing on the shoulders of those who came before you. We are proud to share some of their stories!

We urge you to continue this legacy by sharing your stories with others...

Celebrating Nursing!

Intro: The Essence of Nursing *Margarita Baggett*   173

The Art of Nursing
10 Tips for the New Grad World *Jennifer Perisho*   179
Trusting Your Instincts *Sally Morgan*   180
What Being a Nurse is Really About *Kimberly C. Horton*   182
One Precious Life *Megan Quinn*   184
The Art of Assessment *Daman Mott*   186
Breaking Through the "Difficult" Façade *Sara Glass*   188
Building Your Brain Sheets *Chris Poole*   190
Was I Never Meant to be a Nurse? *Gwen Matthews*   192
Live, Laugh, Holy Crap! *Andrea Natelborg*   194
Give Yourself Time to Learn *Ginger Manss*   196

Our Patients: Forever in Our Hearts
Easing a Patient's Difficult Journey *Karen Price-Gharzeddine*   200
Making the Human Connection *Donna Kistler*   202
Learning from Our Patients *Richard Brock*   204
The Other Patient *Katelyn Clark*   208
The Best, Worst Experience *Heaven Holdbrooks*   210
The First Farewell *Joyce Eden*   212
Caring for My Wounded Brothers and Sisters *Julian Gallegos*   214
It's Much More than Technical Skills *Laura Giambattista*   219

Our Preceptors and Mentors
The Blessing of My Preceptor *Debra Brady*   226
Nothing is as Bad as It Seems *Kelly Navarro*   228
Finding Your Lifeline *Kay Evans*   230
Building Your Competence While Growing Confidence   232
Lourdes C. Salandanan
Was It Early Just Culture? *Robyn Nelson*   234
What Would Florence Do? *Mercy Popoola*   236
Even New Grads Can Take Charge *Jennifer M. Friedenbach*   239

The Health Care Team: Together We're Stronger

The Nerve Center Chris Poole 244
The Art of Listening Peggy Diller 246
Staying Positive Through Adversity Suzette Cardin 248
Better Care Through Effective Teams Kathy Harren 250
Message on My Lunch Bag Kathy Cocking 252
Taking Care of Each Other Bridget Parsh 253

Finding Your Path

The Sweetest Profession of All Kendra Bartlow 257
Nursing: It's My Calling Susan Herman 258
Beginning My Journey Sandra K. Davis 261
When You Know, You Know Kendall Quick 262
The Question Allison Greene 264
Forging New Paths Carrie Garland 266
My "Almost" First Nursing Job Alison Riggs 268
Taking Control of Your Career Jeremy Weed 270
Designing Your Road Map for Success Veanne O'Neill 272
Dreams Beth Gardner 274

The Art of Nursing

"Nursing is my identity, in fact, my obsession!"

Margretta Styles, EdD, RN, FAAN

10 Tips for the New Grad World

As a nurse you're often holding another person's life in your hands. But as a new grad, you're not always sure what to do with it!

I've always held myself to the highest standard. So the transition from senior nursing student to shell-shocked new nurse was a little hard for me to handle. But with the help of some amazing preceptors and supportive family, I made it through.

Looking back on my experience, there are some things I wish I had known sooner rather than later:

- On your first day, you're going to be overwhelmed.
- Don't ever be afraid to ask questions.
- Try to focus on one thing at a time.
- Learn from your mistakes – don't fixate on them.
- Talk to other members of the health care team (doctors, respiratory therapists, pharmacists). You'll be surprised at how much you'll learn.
- Take care of yourself and know your limits.
- It's okay to ask for help – everybody needs it sometimes.
- As a nurse you have a voice, so use it.
- Take time to appreciate the job you're doing, even if it feels like no one else does.
- Even on your busiest days, remember to treat your patients with the love and respect they deserve. It will be a more rewarding experience for everyone.

As an RN, I'm grateful to have a career I love. Even though I still need to remind myself of these tips from time-to-time, when I look back at how much I've grown from my first day on the unit to today, I'm very proud of what I've accomplished.

And trust me, it's all worth it!

Jennifer Perisho, BSN, RN, CCRN
Graduated 2009

Nursing: it's all worth it!

Trusting Your Instincts

My first job was in a labor and delivery unit in a major medical center in New York City. I had just graduated from an associate of arts degree nursing program in Pueblo, Colorado and decided at the age of 19 to try my luck in the Big Apple.

After an intense six-month orientation in labor and delivery, post partum and the newborn nursery, I was caring for low-risk patients in the labor area. This was before the advent of fetal monitors, and I had become reasonably competent at listening to fetal heart tones using a fetascope. Usually, you could only hear the fetal heart tones between contractions, but I decided to listen during a patient's contraction. To my shock, the heart rate severely dropped and seemed to take an unusual amount of time to recover.

I called in the obstetrician and told him what had happened. I listened again with the next contraction and the same bradycardia scenario occurred. The MD looked me in the eye and asked, "Are you sure?"

So many doubts ran through my mind. *Am I not really hearing the bradycardia?* I will look foolish and incompetent if they do a Cesarean section and there is nothing wrong. But I trusted my assessment, and my gut feeling was that something was wrong. So I said, "I'm sure!"

The mother and baby were rushed to the OR for an emergency C-section and a normal baby boy, pink and healthy was born. The obstetrician took me with him to see the father and said, "This nurse just saved your baby's life. She was able to listen to his heartbeat during the contraction and told me it was severely low. Your baby had the cord wrapped tightly around his arms and legs. If labor would have continued, he would be in serious trouble."

The father cried, hugged me and even tried to give me money. I was crying, too. I politely thanked him, and suggested he donate the money to the pediatric toy fund. I touched something very sacred that day, something nurses have the opportunity to be a part of nearly every day.

Forty years later, a labor and delivery nurse and an on-call obstetrician enacted a similar scenario, only with a fetal monitor to guide them instead of a fetascope. Because of their assessment skills and trusting their gut feeling, my grandson was born healthy.

Sally Morgan, PhD, RN
Graduated 1971

Trust yourself and listen to your inner voice!

What Being a Nurse is Really About

When I began my career as a nurse, I was very careful to be methodical and strategic. My end goal was to become a staff nurse in the pediatric intensive care unit (PICU). I possessed a tremendous love for people, particularly the little ones, and simply wanted to be there to make a difference during one of the most vulnerable periods of life – illness.

I first worked in a newborn nursery to learn to care for well babies. I was then afforded an opportunity to participate in a new nurse intensive care training program. This was my chance to learn to care for critically ill adults. The goal was to use my experience and training in critical care to eventually be the best PICU nurse possible. My ICU training program lasted 12 months and I successfully completed it, learning to care for both medical and surgical intensive care patients. Now was my chance to reach my ultimate goal. I applied for and was hired into my first job as a PICU nurse. What a rush I felt. I had reached my goal.

My first two weeks on the job were typical: hospital orientation (my least favorite period), followed immediately by my unit-based orientation (my second least favorite period). Finally I was on my own, independently caring for my patients. My first patient was, as I thought at the time, pretty straight forward: a 3 year-old male, with a history of skeletal contortion. He had been back from the OR for about three hours. The surgeons had taken one of his ribs and placed it along his trachea so that the skeletal contortion did not twist to the point of compromising his airway. My orders were to keep him sedated with Versed and do chest percussions on the operative side every three hours to prevent him from developing pneumonia.

Being the excited, yet particular nurse that I was, I set about to ensure this little guy did not develop pneumonia while under my care. As I prepared to carry out my first round of chest percussions, I followed all procedures, drawing up the Versed and checking it with a second nurse to ensure the dose was correct. I turned him on his side, letting him know what I was going to do. I did all of the things I had been taught to do in nursing school and in my internship. I sedated him and began the chest percussions. I was so diligent in doing my best to prevent this little guy from getting pneumonia.

For some reason (to this day I don't know why) something told me to look at this baby's face. I was so focused on his chest that I wasn't paying attention to the whole person. As I moved my eyes from his chest to his face, I realized that he had tears streaming from his left eye. I couldn't understand how this could be. I had sedated him. How could he be crying? It made no sense. I realized that, although I had given him Versed, I had under-medicated him. He needed more than I had given him. He could feel what I was doing, but wasn't conscious enough to cry out.

My heart sank. It was at that moment I realized I was so focused on the task, that I had forgotten to focus on the person whom the task was meant to help. I had lost sight of the personhood of this little boy.

This was the day I truly understood what being a nurse was about. It was not about the task, but about the person. It was about being there to comfort and protect this person during the most frightening and vulnerable time of his life. It was about making sure he was warm, comfortable and without anxiety. It was about ensuring he recovered, yes, but also that he was at peace and did not suffer any undue stress during an already stressful experience. I had failed him! And this I would never forget!

Each day as you go into your workplaces, never forget the huge responsibility of your role as RNs. To care for, comfort and protect each and every patient – every day, in every encounter. That is what being a nurse is truly about.

Kimberly C. Horton, DHA, MSN, FNP, RN, FACHE
Graduated 1987

Nursing is NOT about the task…it's about the person!

One Precious Life

Through my RN residency program, I've seen and done quite a bit. I placed NG tubes, drew my own labs, made several IV attempts, helped with admissions, observed brain surgery and fed more stubborn babies than I can count. After each shift, as I attempted to de-stress from a hard night's work, I would usually take time to analyze my feelings about the night. But the way I thought about myself as a nurse changed after I took care of Lily.

Lily's case was a difficult one. She had a rough history – a mother who had made some mistakes, and a father who was no longer in the picture. Lily's mother was brought to the hospital under CPR, and was coded throughout Lily's delivery. Barely alive, Lily was placed on brain cooling therapy quickly after she was born, in hopes that the damage to her brain from such a long time with little or no oxygen would be reduced. While Lily was fighting for life, her mother lost her own battle, and Lily became an orphan.

That's when I met Lily. She was a day and a half old and so adorable, even with all her equipment. She didn't do much that first night, but I could sense that I was becoming attached to her. The smallest thing, from the spontaneous opening of one eye to a slight withdrawal from pain, was a huge milestone for her. When I cared for Lily a second night, this time off the brain cooling therapy, watching for those small neurological changes became my mission. I knew her outcome would be unhappy regardless of any left arm movement or Babinski reflex, but I wanted to hold out hope for her. To give her and us something to strive for, just as we do with all our other babies. She didn't have to know about custody battles and that she was named after a mother who would never hold her, she just had to move one baby step at a time.

After taking care of Lily, really taking care of her – combing her hair, watching her behavior, trying to get her to grasp my fingers – I discovered that I felt more like a nurse than ever before. It wasn't just about a series of tasks to be completed, it was about this baby and her life, both now and in the future. I will never forget her story, or the way her tiny fingers wrapped around mine just once, but once nonetheless.

Megan Quinn, BSN, RN
Graduated 2009

Take time to reflect on the lives you've touched!

The Art of Assessment

After graduating from nursing school, I paid my dues as a cardio-pulmonary telemetry nurse for a year. I then applied, interviewed and was accepted on the neuro-trauma unit. I was going to be a trauma/critical care nurse!

I diligently listened to my preceptor. I read everything about neuro and the nervous system I could get my hands on. I attended every critical care class the hospital offered, even on my days off. I asked the doctors questions everyday. For six weeks I followed my preceptor and every other nurse around like a puppy-dog to get every different experience imaginable while I was on orientation.

I practiced my neuro assessment skills until I could do them in my sleep, and I waited with baited breath until I could finally be "alone" to do them all by myself. I had learned that to do them properly you had to be loud. Neuro patients sometimes had cognitive impairments and at times their level of sedation or injury was such that you had to shout to get them to respond to even simple commands.

I was so excited when my first "solo" day arrived. I sat through report as giddy as a school girl. I was fidgety and could barely contain my excitement. I was a little disappointed when the charge nurse assigned me a long-time resident of the unit for my first patient. He had multiple issues including a tracheostomy that prevented him from getting placement in another facility. He bounced frequently from the ortho-uro floor because of non-compliance. The ICU would tune him up and send him back. He had been at the hospital for years. I'll call him Larry.

The charge nurse then told me I would get the first admission. I was a little disheartened, but at least I would be assigned the first admit. Until then, I had to prove myself worthy. I was anxious to join the ranks of the "regular" staff and be unencumbered by a preceptor checking on my every move.

I almost ran from the report room. I did a compulsory sweep of the chart to make sure there were no orders, and then I charged into the room. I did a quick sweep of the pumps and fluids. Was everything in order? Check. I grabbed a step stool and began my head-to-toe assessment. Pupils, facial nerves, soft-sharp, I was getting it done!

I placed my index and middle fingers together and put them in Larry's corresponding palms and gave the command, "Squeeze my fingers." Nothing.

Undaunted I raised my voice and said loudly, "Come on Larry, you can do it, squeeze my fingers." Nothing.

Not wanting to fail, I was almost shouting, "Larry, Larry, squeeze my fingers!"

Larry looked up at me and in a voice I'll never forget said, "I'm a quad you ass!"

I felt terrible and the laughter that erupted was deafening. I turned to see all my co-workers standing in the doorway to Larry's room and Larry was laughing as hard as any of them. I stormed off the unit as embarrassed as could be.

I learned an important lesson that stays with me to this day: take what you do seriously, but don't take yourself too seriously!

Daman Mott, MSN, RN
Graduated 1999

When assessing your patients, always consider the unique individual before you.

Breaking Through the "Difficult" Facade

During nursing school there's so much information to absorb that it's hard to imagine there's anything you didn't already learn. However, as soon as you set foot in the hospital as a registered nurse, you realize just how wrong you were. During my first few months as an RN, I've learned so much about myself and how to be a nurse as I provide care for my patients and their families.

On one particular shift, I cared for a one year-old baby girl who was accompanied by her mother. They had been admitted in the middle of the night, and had been given few answers about possible diagnoses, testing needed and how long the admission might be. When I entered the room at the beginning of my shift, it was clear that the mom was very scared and desperate for information about her daughter's condition. After answering her immediate questions and completing my morning assessment, I informed her that I would find out more details about her daughter's plan of care from the doctor.

Fortunately the next time I entered the room, I was able to provide the mother with much more information. She was very grateful and much less anxious. Throughout the day, when I went into this patient's room, I made sure to take the time to give the mom the information and support she so desperately needed. By spending this extra time, I discovered that the mom was in the process of getting a divorce, received little support from her extended family and her daughter was her first successful pregnancy after seven miscarriages. She was terrified of losing her only child. Needless to say, her anxiety was understandable when put in the context of her personal life.

Since I was returning for a second shift the following day, I was again assigned to care for this patient and her mother. I was careful to organize my day in a way that would allow me to spend extra time with this family when needed. After conducting several tests, the doctors found that everything was normal and the baby was prepared for discharge. When discharge instructions were completed, the mom gave me a huge hug and said: "Thank you. I don't think I could have emotionally made it through these last two days without you!"

At that moment, I remembered very vividly why I became a nurse: I want to care for and support families as they experience the most scary and challenging times in their lives.

My time as an RN resident has provided a safe environment to help me learn and grow in my role as a nurse. Now that I feel more comfortable with the procedural side of nursing, I have the time and freedom to provide family-centered care to each of my patients and their families. I've learned that being a good nurse doesn't mean I simply do my work flawlessly, but that I can be the difference between a miserable hospitalization and a peaceful one. Now that I've seen this play out in my own personal practice, there's no turning back.

Sara Glass, BSN, RN, CPN
Graduated 2010

Nurses frame difficult conversations to show support and understanding.

Building Your Brain Sheets

As a new nurse getting report with my preceptor, I was completely blown away by how the more experienced nurses could take in large amounts of information, much of the time without even writing it down. I work on a medical/surgical unit with a nurse/patient ratio of 5:1. Those are five patients, each with IVs, BMs, extensive medical histories, labs to draw and the list goes on.

It was like getting 10 minutes of driving directions in a foreign city: turn left at *Colostomy Way*, right at the *PICC Change*, past the *500 ml Bladder Scan at 0400* – and don't forget to stop for *Crackles in the Right Lower Lobe....*

I came to realize that the brain, once exposed to an important category of information over and over, creates a method of storage like a little box. That box might be called "past medical history" or "allergies," and it's in your head even when empty, just waiting to be filled. With time, instead of a huge mass of random data, you have a tidy place to put everything.

A box, just like the ones we have on our brain sheets.

Think for a minute about getting directions in a city, but imagine that it's your home city. You have a map in your head and you can see the route being described to you.

A brain sheet is a reflection of our own brain. Are you the type of nurse who uses four colors of ink and writes in a miniscule font? Or one that prints out two full pages of information on each of your patients and then makes notes in the margins? I knew an excellent nurse who never wrote down a single letter, not even an occasional set of vitals on an alcohol swab package. As new nurses, I think the process of creating our brain sheets and developing our actual nursing brain go hand-in-hand, both influencing the other.

So with the very precious time you have as a new grad, make a brain sheet of your own. I used an old-fashioned pencil, ruler and eraser. I asked my wife's computer-savvy sister to re-create it on the computer. Then, I had 100 copies made, front and back.

Review the sheets you've used (then shred them to maintain confidentiality). See which boxes you filled consistently and which ones weren't used. Then, reformat your sheet accordingly.

Take it from me, you'll be doing more than just looking well prepared. You'll be reinforcing those boxes in your brain and creating a nursing road map to help you navigate your clinical practice.

Chris Poole, BSN, RN
Graduated 2010

Develop your system to organize your work and learning.

Was I Never Meant to be a Nurse?

Decades ago, I graduated during a nursing shortage and had the good fortune of being hired directly into critical care.

At that time there were no formalized training programs, articulated competencies or didactic sessions other than passing the cardiac test through the American Heart Association. Instead, I went into an apprentice role, shadowing a more experienced nurse.

Just a couple of months into my employment, I already had my own patient assignment and began to hang a Pronestyl drip for a patient. In those days we did not have pumps, so I set and adjusted the administration by counting the drops per minute in the drip chamber and calculating the rate of infusion. Minutes after the infusion began, I was dismayed to see the patient's blood pressure plummet and their color change. I quickly stopped the infusion to see if that was the causative factor.

As I quickly glanced over the setup, I saw that I had inadvertently hung macro drip tubing rather than micro drip tubing, resulting in a delivery volume four times what I had intended. In my haste to quickly and effectively treat the patient, I had made a medication error via my choice of tubing.

I was devastated! I remembered hearing about a patient who had died as a result of a nurse making the very same error, and realized how close I had come. Thoughts of self-recrimination raced through my mind: "How could I have been so careless? I could have killed that person! I don't deserve to be a nurse!"

In the midst of that experience, I resolved to make patient safety my first priority, so I would never have to feel that way again. The weighty responsibility of having a life entrusted into my care was indelibly etched in my heart and mind. I resolved to be the best nurse I could be, learning everything I possibly could, being ultra-attentive to each aspect of my care, and enjoining others if I was undertaking a high-risk task. I thanked God that my learning had not been at the expense of a patient's life.

This experience made such a profound impact on me. I am thankful I didn't give up nursing at the time. It has been a deeply rewarding profession every step of the way.

Gwen Matthews, MSN, MBA, RN
Graduated 1975

We all make mistakes – we need to learn from our own and each other's.

Live, Laugh, Holy Crap!

As I stand at the gas pump filling my tank, my mind wanders and I think of death and dying. Everyone in this world has the opportunity to meet death one day, and I am suddenly worried about not doing everything I want to do in life.

The gas pump beeps, and I'm alive. I'm suddenly filled with warmth and happiness. I am alive and I'm so grateful.

Live! *Random House Dictionary* defines being alive as "having life; living; existing." Many of my patients on the pediatric oncology unit wish for life. They are fighting an ongoing battle to live each and every day. So many of us take life for granted. We are blessed to be alive and healthy. To have the faith that tomorrow morning we will rise and the day will pass with another on its way.

Life is such a wonderful gift. Working in oncology has furthered my appreciation of life. Everywhere I go, I see an opportunity to share life and happiness with someone else. My hope is to touch a life, even if it's in a small way, and make it better.

Laugh! Laughing is all we seem to do on my oncology unit. Laughing helps lift our spirits. Getting a sick kid to laugh is like the lights on my Christmas tree – breathtaking and mood lifting. Sweet faces smiling at me fill my heart with warmth. Parents saying thank-you and giving hugs provide the sheer satisfaction that I am making a difference.

Many people hear oncology, and quickly say, "Oh that's so sad." Sad it definitely is, but it can be happy too. Our kids have sharp personalities. They are quick, witty and have the best attitudes. Recently during a procedure, I had a teen patient who wouldn't settle down enough to allow his medications to relax him. We were just about to start his bone marrow biopsy when he said in a groggy voice, "Wait! I'm still awake!" We all looked at each other and tried not to giggle. He was 17 and had done this many times before. The medications given would cause him to have amnesia and also not to feel any pain, but he was still able to talk.

Later that day, he was thanking me for helping him during the procedure. He was such a kind and polite young man. I told him that he was quite a character in the procedure room. To my relief, he couldn't remember the procedure, but he eagerly wanted to know what he had said or done. I related how he insisted he was awake and needed more medication. We all laughed and his mom was happy to be part of the story.

HOLY CRAP!! Blood Pressure 77/42! Okay I think to myself: stay calm, don't panic. Retake the blood pressure...then panic! My patient was crashing and I was the first on the scene. I told my patient's dad that her blood pressure was a little low and I was going to give her some extra fluid in her "tubies" to help raise it.

Along with my preceptor, Karen, we paged the doctor on call with our patient's status. Karen had two, one liter bags of normal saline and was filling 60 ml syringes one after the other and handing them to me. I had the job of pushing the fluid through the IV tubing which seemed like the diameter of a toothpick.

The goal is to slam the fluid in! Slam? I was sweating, my thumbs were throbbing from pushing and my patient was crying. After pushing 1,140 mls of fluid into my little patient, the physician decided she should be transferred to the ICU where she could be put on a dopamine drip.

My patient did wonderfully! She walked up to me five days later and said "hi" with her sweet smile. Her dad was very grateful and thanked me for everything. I was so happy and proud of myself. My "holy crap" moment became a "holy crap I'm good" moment. I had made it, and so had my patient. My support group that day and everyday on the oncology unit is what keeps bringing me back to work each week. I love the kids! They're the foundation that gives me the strength and desire to grow into the best nurse possible.

Andrea Natelborg, BSN, RN
Graduated 2010

We all need support at times. Be part of the team – they are your foundation!

Give Yourself Time to Learn

I've been a nurse for decades, but still recall with vivid clarity one particular day when I had been working on my oncology unit for about a year.

I admitted a patient with acute myelogenous leukemia who required a significant amount of care. I did his admission assessment, accessed his central line, drew blood cultures, started a transfusion, gave him antibiotics and worked hard to make him comfortable.

About three hours after he arrived on the floor, my patient began having symptoms of septic shock and respiratory distress. I immediately called his doctor, drew stat ABGs, called the respiratory therapist and got orders to transfer him to the ICU.

I distinctly remember my charge nurse walking back from lunch as we were moving the patient, and she asked me what I was doing. I told her that I was transferring my patient to the ICU (this was before the days of rapid response teams). She asked why I didn't call her, and my flippant reply as we wheeled him away was: "Well, because I didn't need you!"

Later that evening as I walked out of the hospital, I thought to myself: *Wow, I gave great care today,* and congratulated myself as I reviewed my day. Then it hit me like a ton of bricks! If this was the first day of giving absolutely great care, what in the world had I been doing with every other patient I cared for in the past year? Had I given mediocre care? I must have! I felt terrible!

It took quite a bit of introspection to realize that during my first year I had worked very hard and tried to do a good job, but my best was not *the* best. I came to realize that each day in nursing you can only give your very best to the patient in front of you – whatever your best may be at this stage in your career.

My advice for new nurses is this: be true to yourself, honor the fact that you need to learn, adjust and maximize your skills. Give yourself a break, celebrate the things you do right each day and give yourself the *TIME* to become the most effective and special nurse *YOU* can be!

Ginger Manss, MSN, RN, AOCN
2012 ACNL President
Graduated 1982

Always strive to give your best, knowing that as a nurse you will continue to grow.

Our Patients:
Forever In Our Hearts

"*People will forget what you said, people will forget what you did, but people will never forget how you made them feel.*"

Maya Angelou

Easing a Patient's Difficult Journey

I was so excited when I graduated from nursing school! I was thrilled to wear the white starched uniform with white stockings, polished white shoes and clean white shoe laces. I proudly wore my white cap on my head and my nursing pin on my left shoulder.

My first job was on the night shift of a 34-bed oncology unit, working five nights a week with every other weekend off. It felt like heaven to have a career doing what I loved – caring for patients and families.

One of my most memorable experiences as a new grad was caring for Margaret, a 40 year-old college professor. Diagnosed with metastatic bone cancer, Margaret was undergoing chemotherapy and, as a result, was losing her hair in large clumps. Margaret loved poetry, and books of poems lined the window sill of her hospital room. Whenever possible during my shift, I would close the door, sit on Margaret's bed (which you weren't supposed to do!) and I would hold her hand while reading poetry to her.

Margaret had difficulty sleeping because of the excruciating pain she experienced, so I tried to make her as comfortable as possible. Margaret's appearance was very important to her. She wore red nail polish that was neatly manicured. I would often help her apply her makeup. To hide the hair loss that resulted from chemotherapy, Margaret would wear beautiful scarves.

I was deeply moved by Margaret's strength as she battled her illness. On several occasions, she emphasized how important it is to be caring and compassionate and urged me not lose sight of this. Throughout my career, Margaret's words have stayed with me.

One weekend, I bought Margaret a book written by one of her favorite authors. I was so excited to give it to her on Monday. When I went to her room before my shift started, I found the room empty and set up for a new patient. I walked quickly to the desk and asked where she had been moved to. The charge nurse took me into a conference room and broke the news that Margaret had passed away over the weekend. I was devastated and began crying. The charge nurse held me tightly and said to always remember how I touched Margaret's heart and provided compassionate care during her last days on earth.

I'll always remember this patient and how she touched my life. I share this story with new graduates whenever possible to emphasize how we as nurses make a difference to others. Although it has been many years since my first job as a nurse, I still take great pride in our profession and am very thankful that I found my calling at a young age.

If I may share some words of wisdom: Ignite your passion as you find your calling in nursing. No matter where your career takes you, always strive to provide quality, compassionate care.

Karen Price-Gharzeddine, BSN, MS, RN
2013 ACNL President
Graduated 1980

Never lose sight of the caring and compassionate side of nursing!

Making the Human Connection

One memorable summer night as a new grad, I was receiving a post-op patient in the ICU who had suffered a recent trauma. Sam was in his early twenties, and had survived a diving accident that unfortunately left him quadriplegic. I immediately began my assessment while rehearsing in my mind what I needed to do for this young man.

Sam was the same age as me and now he was a quadriplegic. I couldn't imagine it! I utilized my nursing knowledge to stay focused on caring for him throughout the shift. On the nights that followed, I was often assigned to be Sam's nurse. After delivering the best nursing care I could, I decided to get to know him better so that I could try to address his emotional needs. I learned that great care happens when one human being truly connects with another.

One night Sam was able to talk about the accident. He was visiting the area with friends and having a great vacation until they decided to go diving in some "risky" areas of the lake. "We were all enjoying diving into the water until I dove in and hit a rock," Sam explained. "Then I realized I couldn't move. I was so scared."

After the trauma of being brought to the hospital with no feeling in his arms or legs, Sam became dependent on the hospital staff for his every need. While caring for him, Sam became my central focus. I was determined to assist him in achieving his maximum potential. He loved to talk, and would wait for me (the avid listener) to arrive on the night shift so I could hear about the events of his day. It was so special when Sam told me he would try to sleep during the day so he could be awake when I came on duty. That way, we would have more time to talk. I learned that healing is definitely maximized when patients feel safe and cared for.

I felt honored caring for Sam and getting to know him during this tragic time in his life. We connected as nurse and patient, and I was able to give him honest feedback, encouragement and above all, hope. When Sam left our unit for rehab, I visited him and followed his progress until discharge. Sam did quite well and learned all the strategies to manage his quadriplegia.

But wait, the story doesn't end there!

A few years later, I was working in another hospital as an assistant manager in a nearby city. I was receiving report when I learned my new patient for the day would be Sam! I was now working in Sam's hometown and he was being admitted to my unit.

Imagine his surprise when he discovered I was his nurse! Since the last time I saw him, Sam had become quite independent and had a caregiver by his side. We were able to catch up on the past and once again resumed our nurse-patient relationship.

I found it so rewarding to inform the treatment team of Sam's progress and his care from the initial diving injury. Once again, I was able to connect with him as a patient and a person and deliver the care he needed.

It is paramount that we treat all patients with kindness, compassion and respect while genuinely making human connections with the people entrusted in our care. And now 35 years later as a seasoned nurse leader, I will always remember caring for Sam and the impact he had on me as a new nurse.

Donna Kistler, MS, RN
2008 ACNL President
Graduated 1977

Healing is maximized when patients feel safe and cared for.

Learning from Our Patients...

One nurse's story about two very memorable patients.

The Story of Bunny Hare

I was a new graduate and still on orientation at my first job as a staff nurse. I was working on a 55-bed male surgical ward – the old kind of ward with 55 beds all lined up with only thin curtains separating each patient. There was no privacy, and in those days there was no such thing as a "HIPAA violation." The Joint Commission would have had a ball citing HIPAA violations since everything a caregiver said and did to or with a patient was overheard by many beyond those flimsy curtains.

As a recent graduate and a real RN, I didn't want to do or say something that could be construed by anyone as anything but professional, appropriate, therapeutic and even brilliant.

This particular day, I was assigned to care for William Hare (not his real name), a post-operative patient who had surgery for removal of a cancerous growth on his left earlobe. Today, the procedure would likely have been done as outpatient surgery, but in the 1960s, the procedure required admission for pre-op tests the night before the surgery, at least a day in the hospital on the day of surgery, with anticipation of discharge the day after surgery. The reason William Hare is outstanding in my memory is that he was so wise, and at 103 years old, he was the oldest person I had ever seen!

Before I met the patient, I dreaded having to take care of someone so ancient. What do you say to someone who is 103 when you are in your early 30s?

Here's the conversation we had:

Nurse (me): (speaking loudly) Good morning, Mr. Hare. Do you like to be called Mr. or do you prefer William or Bill?

Patient: You don't have to yell. And I don't prefer any of those names. They call me Bunny.

Nurse: Well, alright, Bunny. I suppose they call you Bunny because your last name is Hare, right?

Patient: You're smart, young man – very smart.

Nurse: So, Bunny – what brought you to the hospital? (in school, they told us that was always a good ice-breaker question).

Patient: A 1958 Chevy Impala – it was driven by my 82 year old son, in case that's your next question.

Nurse: That's very interesting, Bunny. (long pause while I get the pan of water, a towel and washcloth in place) So, I see from your chart that you are 103 years old?

Patient: Nope. Actually, I'm 103 plus 10 months and I think about two more weeks if you're really counting.

Nurse: That's really wonderful!

Patient: Really? I never gave it too much thought.

Nurse: Well, so – (now my brilliance is really beginning to shine!) tell me, Bunny, how does a person get to be 103?

Patient: (after a long pause and an amazed stare at me) Well first off, you go to bed every night. Then you get up the next morning. Then, that night, you go to bed once again. The next morning you get up again. That night – are you beginning to see a pattern here, son? That night, you go to bed again. The most important part of all this is that you get up again the next morning. And here's the secret – if you do it enough times, you too, young man, can get to be 103!

Well, I haven't reached it yet, but I've been following Bunny's advice for years now, and I am making progress!

The Story of Tootsie

I was working the day shift as a staff RN in a cardio-pulmonary unit in a New York City medical center. Our unit did thoracotomies, cardiac bypasses, general surgery and many pacemakers and battery changes.

Tootsie was in her late 80s and originally from the Ukraine. She was a retired high-fashion cosmetician. She was bright and spoke with a slight accent. According to Tootsie, her client list included some of the world's most beautiful women. Tootsie's own make-up made her look 30 years younger (if you viewed her from a distance). She was really quite glamorous.

Tootsie was admitted to my unit for her third pacemaker battery replacement. According to Tootsie, "I live life so fast, the batteries just can't keep up with me!"

I did Tootsie's initial interview and assessment when she was admitted to my floor one day prior to having the procedure. The interview went something like this:

Question: "Your date of birth"
Answer: "Not a question a gentleman asks a lady."

Question: "What medications do you take on a regular basis?"
Answer: "Two martinis before dinner and a brandy before bed."

I found her responses unique and her whole outlook on life invigorating!

When I tried to do Tootsie's individualized care plan, this is what she told me: "*Dahlink*, I only wish one *think* on my caring plan – have the girls [nurses] wake me at five each *mornink* so I put on my face before the boys [doctors] walk around!" (Remember, Tootsie was a dedicated cosmetician!).

Tootsie's focus on make-up was emphasized one afternoon when I overheard a conversation in her room from the hallway. Her roommate (a forty-year old post-op) was moaning and groaning. I was in the process of seeing if this patient would like something for pain when I heard Tootsie say:

Dahlink – you must not whimper and whine like this. Do you not see that a whine makes valleys and caverns in the face that even a plastic surgeon cannot excavate. Even I cannot repair the damage you make on the face with my creams, lotions and salves.

Do your face a favor, my *dahlink* – when you feel a wince *comink* on, push upon the little button that says "call light." The nurse then comes and gives relief pills that make your face beautiful!

Because the night shift nurses woke Tootsie promptly at 5 a.m. each morning before the doctors rounded, Tootsie called me her *"Prime Nurse."* (We were trying to do primary nursing in those days). I tried to give Tootsie discharge instructions: how to take her pulse, signs of pacemaker battery failure and phone numbers to call in case of emergency. She listened to me patiently for a while, then patted my hand, saying: "Pause, please. You do this *Prime Nurse* job very good, but I must say to you this – I don't need to know these *thinks* – I do not need the numbers on the phone or the very important *thinks* you are telling me. My nephew is my doctor and he lives right next door in my *buildink*. If I have trouble, my cane I tap on the wall and *presto-zingo*, he comes to my rescue – every time!"

When Tootsie was discharged, she asked for me to be the one who wheeled her to the lobby. On the way, she secretly handed me an envelope. "For you because you are special *Prime Nurse* to me."

After she left, I opened the envelope. It was a Christmas card (even though this was mid-July) and she wrote, "Too busy to shop but I love you and your caring to me – *Tootsie*." Enclosed in the card was a wrinkled one-dollar bill. I don't think I ever received a gift more genuinely given.

Richard Brock, BSN, BA, MA, RN, NEA-BC
1994 ACNL President
Graduated 1969

When we take the time to listen, we can learn so much from our patients.

The Other Patient

When I decided to become a nurse, I had no idea which area of nursing I wanted to practice. When asked, I would always reply: "I'm not really sure, but I will never go into pediatrics!"

Imagine my surprise when I loved my pediatric rotation. Although I had found my niche in pediatrics, I was warned by colleagues that pediatric patients are great to care for, but the parents are the "patients" who can be difficult.

With this in mind, I began my career in pediatrics excited, anxious and terrified all at the same time. Throughout my time in the PICU there have been crazy days, mellow days and more crazy days. Despite this, one of my daily goals remained the same: to recognize that there is a child in the hospital bed, and sitting across from them is our other patient – the parent.

I've realized that for every resilient kid we care for, there is a terrified parent who deserves our best care too. Although these kids are so sick, I feel a certain peace knowing that, as nurses, we're doing our best to control their pain and make them comfortable. My heart bleeds for the parents who look upon their child with a sense of nervous helplessness.

In these moments, I feel empathy for these parents. I feel a connection with them, not because I have kids, or have even come close to being in their shoes. I think it's because in the midst of a busy day full of orders, medications, assessments and charting, I have felt overwhelmed and even helpless at times, but thankful to have a preceptor and helpful coworkers to turn to for guidance.

Ultimately, I want to provide guidance and support for these parents, always remembering that often the parents suffer just as much as the patients themselves.

Katelyn Clark, BSN, RN, CCRN
Graduated 2010

Never forget that your patient is part of a family – as nurses we care for them all.

The Best, Worst Experience

Just four months into my first job as a new grad, I learned and experienced more of what being a nurse truly means than during my entire four years in college. I learned that every day I work as an RN, I'm here for a purpose. I'm here for the children – to help a patient, parent or family have the best experience possible in the worst situation of their lives.

And just as I have the chance to dramatically impact the lives of others, I'm constantly touched and changed by the patients and families I care for. One family and patient in particular I will never forget.

I arrived at work on what seemed to be a typical Tuesday – alarms beeping, drips running, ventilator pistons making loud vibrating noises, medications being administered and tasks to be completed before the shift even began. My assigned patient was a premature two-week old infant who was born at 23 weeks and hanging onto life by a thread. Sadly, she had been diagnosed with bilateral grade four bleeds with no chance of recovery. Today, the doctors were going to break the news to the parents and suggest we take their baby off life support. All the machines, drips and lines seemed to disappear with the realization that a little life was underneath all of the chaos.

The members of the health care team, including me, were going to break the worst news of a parent's lifetime – that their child was not going to survive. Any bad day I've ever had was thrown out the window. I could only imagine the pain, sorrow and heartbreak these parents would feel. I wished there was something more we could do, but we had exhausted all possible options and the prognosis for the baby was irreversible. I knew the only thing I could do was to try and give the parents the best, worst experience of their lives.

After breaking the news to the parents, we gave them as much time as they needed to consider the decision to remove their baby from life support. Ultimately it had to be the parents' decision. No matter what my own personal views were or what the health care team thought was right, the parents would be the ones to live with their decision for the rest of their lives.

After many tears, bringing in other family members, talking to the parents' local doctor for a second opinion and explaining the prognosis several times to each family member, the parents and family made a decision. They made one of the hardest decisions of their lives – to let their baby go, because they wanted what was best for their child. We made sure to accommodate the family as best we could during this difficult time. Throughout the shift, I had a flood of emotions and my heart went out to the parents. I knew I had to not only give the best care to their daughter, but also to the family. I wanted to do all I could for them.

This was a day I will never forget. It will constantly remind me that behind all of the machines, noise, lines and chaos of the NICU, there is a child, a human being whose life depends on the care I give. I have the rare opportunity every day to impact a family's life and to leave them with memories they will hold onto for the rest of their lives. To me this makes being a nurse worth every moment.

Being a nurse is more than just a job – it is a way of life!

Heaven Holdbrooks, BSN, RN
Graduated 2010

RNs know the clinical procedure side thoroughly, but make a real difference connecting with patients on the caring side.

The First Farewell

He had wasted away to skin and bones from his cancer. His wife celebrated a spoonful of broth passing his lips. This was a lesson then and for the future about how small acts of routine activity can be comforting for the family.

Mr. S was trying to be so brave for everyone around him. He would attempt to eat thinking that if he could get his strength back, he could go home. Each bite would set off audible stomach gurgling. (I better understood why bowel sounds had been named borborigamy and never forgot this unusual word). I tried every imaginable food that qualified as a soft or liquid diet to get him to eat. It was my responsibility after all, as the RN on duty, to make sure the nutrition part of his care plan was met. Then there was the pain control part of the care plan. What was I doing asking him to eat when it triggered visible and audible pain for him?

Mr. and Mrs. S had been married for nearly 50 years. They were the kind of couple who could read each other's eyes and finish each other's sentences. As I got to know them over the two weeks I was privileged to care for Mr. S – it was very apparent that he and his wife had a very strong spiritual foundation. I couldn't help but listen in as I came and went to deliver care. I felt most fortunate that I had been trained in patient-centered care long before it had that official title.

I had been raised as a missionary kid in the bush of West Africa. Living with dying was a constant experience, but so was watching those who believed in a heaven. They often died in such peace despite the pain and grief the loss was going to create. I began to inquire what Mr. S really wanted for his care. As we talked about this over the next few days, his wife joined the conversation. He was able to tell her that he had fought the good fight and death held no sting for him.

One evening, I made my last rounds before change of shift. Mr. *S* was in significant pain and agreed to let me administer pain medication. This was prior to PCAs or pain infusion meds on the nursing floors. I gently found a spot on his hip to give him his injection and settled him back in a position that was most comfortable. Through his dry lips he quoted, "*O death where is thy sting? O grave where is thy victory?*"

When I returned the next day, Mr. *S* had been released from the pain of this earth. I stepped into a side hallway to let the tears slide down my face. This was my first farewell to a patient I would grow close to over time. Sometimes I still step away to grieve. At other times, I shed tears with the family.

It is always a loss to say farewell to someone you care about. Being a nurse has allowed me to celebrate that I was there to help, comfort and make a memory that will hopefully be a good and respectful farewell.

Joyce Eden, BS, MHA, RN
Graduated 1980

As nurses we honor our patients' journeys, regardless of where it takes them...

Caring for My Wounded Brothers and Sisters

"Lieutenant Gallegos, you've been selected for deployment!" I will never forget how this one sentence sent my mind into a frenzy. The realization of my duty to my country had in an instant become apparent. Regardless of my own fears, my name had been picked and I had an obligation to my fellow nurses and service members to serve them in the capacity that I had volunteered for only 1½ years previously. Prior to the 9/11 tragedy, I had already decided that upon graduation from nursing school I would join the United States Air Force as an officer and a nurse.

At this point in my career, I was still a new nurse honing my critical thinking and assessment skills. To my benefit, the US Air Force had entrusted to me the lives of its most valued asset – my fellow airmen. Within a short period of time, the military had trained me in leadership and helped build my clinical competence within my profession.

After hearing the sentence that had caused such uneasiness, I took a deep breath and asked where they were sending me. My orders were not to the harsh environments of Iraq or Afghanistan, but to Germany. I had been volunteered by my commander to deploy as a member of a Contingency Aeromedical Staging Facility (CASF). In short, this was the point in the military evacuation system for injured troops coming back from the battlefields for transport to either the local US Army Hopital in Landstuhl, Germany, or for futher care at military health facilities within the United States.

My anxiety at that point subsided somewhat. I knew now that I wasn't going to be risking my life around the battlefields, but helping in the transport and care of my fellow injured brothers and sisters in arms to higher levels of care. I still had some hesitancy about my skills, not because I didn't know what I was doing, but because I would be required to function under totally different circumstances.

The US Air Force prepared us for deployment within a few weeks, and the day after Christmas we were on our flight from San Francisco to Germany. On the flight, I wondered what to expect when we landed.

Within a "short" 14 hours, our group, selected from Travis Air Force Base, landed and was quickly transported via ambulance bus to Ramstein Air Force Base. I remember being exhausted from the flight and arrived at my quarters in the late evening around midnight. I made calls home to notify my family that I had arrived safely. I tried to sleep, since we had been notified that our shift was to begin at 0500 the following day. No chance to recoup from jet lag.

I awoke at 0430 and prepared myself for a long day. I remember walking to the Contingency Aeromedical Staging Facility(CASF) on the base for the first time. The sun obviously was not out and there was a cold breeze that picked up and blew the small amount of snow that had fallen during the night. To think that here I was freezing from the cold in Germany, while my fellow service members were suffering the heat of the Middle East.

I arrived at the CASF and was escorted to the waiting area where typically the injured "walking" troops were debriefed on the process for their transport back to the US. There the group of registered nurses, physicians and medical technicians were briefed on our responsibilities and what our schedules would be. I had been selected for the evening shift, but in the military I knew that really didn't mean anything because you're on-call 24/7.

The first day of deployment was an experience I will never forget. Immediately, another nurse and I were selected to go on a transport that was arriving from Iraq. Along with six medical techs we were shuttled via ambulance bus from the CASF onto the base flight line tarmac to await the arrival of the C-17 transporting patients.

Within minutes the plane landed, and the bus lurched forward to meet it. Once near the back end of the plane, the large hatch lowered creating a gaping hole from which you could see the entire inside or "belly" of the plane. I could see people inside the plane, but couldn't tell much from my vantage point. The hatch served as a ramp and the ambulance bus backed up toward it. These planes are usually used to ship large cargo, but in this plane there were 25-40 injured service members. More than half were able to ambulate off the plane and onto the bus, while the rest were on MASH-style gurneys.

The other nurse and I were directed to accompany one of the flight techs from the plane. We were ushered, not to the gaping hole at the end of the plane, but to a set of stairs on the side of the plane. The technical sergeant was making an attempt to deliver instructions to us, but we couldn't hear because of the running engines. All I could decipher was that we were to seek out the flight nurse onboard so that we could get report.

As I stood at the side of the plane, I could see the side door was open so we made our way up the stairs. I was extremely anxious in anticipation of what was coming next. As I stood at the entrance to the plane, I was immediately made aware of the realities of war. In front of me were eight coffins draped with American flags. These were my fellow service members who hadn't made the trip back home alive. Emotions began to swell, but I knew now was not the time. I needed to do my job. I immediately composed myself as I saw a respiratory tech coming toward us. I asked where the flight nurse was, and he pointed to the stacked gurneys in the middle of the plane.

The flight nurse noticed us coming as she continued to adjust the NG tube for a patient lying on one of the gurneys. We informed her that we were the nurses who were going to accompany the patients to the CASF and Landstuhl Medical Center. She introduced herself and immediately began giving us report on the 25-40 patients, emphasizing only those with major injuries. She handed me their one page medical records describing injury or diagnosis, medications prescribed and administered since the flight from the battlefield, antibiotics due and treatments provided onboard. We then completed a count of all the narcotics that we were taking possession of on behalf of the patients.

After this was completed, we were tasked with assisting in transporting the patients on gurneys to the bus. Within the plane they were stacked three gurneys high, but on the bus we could only stack them by two.

As we transported patients, I could see the pain and confusion on the faces of those who were awake and alert. Many asked questions for which I had no answers, while others said nothing. The "walking" wounded were ushered to the front of the bus where they sat awaiting transport.

Once we loaded the patients, the other RN and I boarded the bus. As the bus door closed behind us, I divided the patient charts between the two of us. I scanned my charts to ascertain which patients needed medications en route to Landstuhl Medical Center.

What was I doing? I was so confused, yet I was expected to react swiftly and make quick, but prudent decisions. The transport to Landstuhl would take approximately 35-40 minutes due to the weather conditions. I triaged which patients needed my immediate attention, and asked the medical technicians to attend to the others.

The first patient I approached had an antibiotic due. I looked at his nametag and confirmed verbally he was the correct patient. I introduced myself and explained to him what I was doing. He happened to be a Marine who had been injured by an improvised explosive device (IED). Only 12 hours prior to his flight to Germany, he had surgery to amputate his left leg above the knee.

I can vividly remember how sincerely he looked up at me, and noticing my rank, he said: "Sir, I am in a lot of pain. I can't stand this any longer, I just want to die."

I let him know that I would give him something for pain. We could utilize standing orders for narcotics as long as the patient had no contraindications. This patient had medication ordered and I was authorized to give him the medication IV or IM. At this point I thought about how much I was going to give him. Our standing orders were significantly general, yet safe in the amount to give. I didn't want to harm him and cause more complications. I utilized my nursing judgment based on my assessment. In the hospital I had the cushion of allowing a physician to make that decision, but now I had the authority to make the decision myself.

I decided to give him 10 mg Morphine IV. I looked at the Marine and told him what I was doing. As I assessed his IV patency, he thanked me for being a nurse. He mentioned that he felt indebted to the US Air Force physicians, nurses and medical technicians who had cared for him in Iraq and were helping him on his journey home. I told him that it was my duty to him as a fellow service member and a human being. IV patency was good as I proceeded to give him the Morphine. Within five minutes, he was feeling much better.

I told him I had other patients to check, but that I would get back to him as soon as I could. I attended to the needs of the other patients, administering antibiotics and narcotics as needed.

The drive to Landstuhl seemed to take forever. As we approached the smaller roads in the drive to the medical center, the ride became bumpier. Patients in the gurneys were swinging back and forth hitting up against the windows. I noticed that the Marine who received the IV Morphine was grimacing again. His gurney was smacking the side of the bus with every bump and I could see that his stump was starting to bleed through its dressing. I asked one of the medical technicians to help me reinforce the dressing and hold pressure. For the remainder of the trip, I held the gurney from hitting up against the side of the bus. The Marine expressed his gratitude, saying he would never forget what we had done for him and that he was proud to serve alongside individuals like us.

We eventually arrived at the medical center where we unloaded the patients. Nursing and medical staff were given report. We gathered the gurneys and made our way back to Ramstein Air Force Base. The shift had just begun and another plane was on its way. On the drive back to the base, I realized why I had chosen nursing as a profession.

From my first day of deployment, I was more eager to help because I discovered that everything I did, even if it seemed insignificant to me, brought comfort to an injured service member. While studying nursing, I never realized the impact I could make in people's lives by being a nurse.

Julian Gallegos, MSN, RN, FNP-BC
Graduated 2001

Rely on your nursing judgement...know your practice and authority.

It's Much More Than Technical Skills

I sat briefly at a computer in the nurse's station. I felt instant relief in my feet as I sank into the plastic computer chair, which at that moment felt like a plush recliner. It was eight hours into my shift with four more to go, and my body was exhausted. My mind continued to race, reviewing all the things I had yet to complete. Change two dressings, discharge a patient, draw labs and coordinate a patient's CT scan.

It was still early in my orientation on a busy medical/surgical floor, and I felt as though I could barely keep up with the day's tasks. Actually it was more like a feeling of drowning. I was out to sea in an ocean of tasks which I wasn't comfortable completing without guidance and supervision. It was a general feeling of incompetence, as if I was in a suspended state of bewilderment and input overload.

Where do we keep that? Where do I chart that? How do I get this IV machine to stop beeping? What's the lab's number? Should I page the doctor for this?

I quickly reviewed orders for a patient and silently hoped that I wouldn't be required to do anything skill-oriented, as this provoked the most stomach tightening anxiety. I sat at the computer in near desperation and prayed to the phantom gods of new nurses: *Dear new nurse gods (and Florence if you're there, too!) please don't make me insert a catheter in an unsuspecting innocent soul, torture someone with an IV insertion attempt or anything of the like. I promise I'll be a good nurse one day, just don't make me do it today!*

These are skills I certainly wanted to acquire, just not right now. It was so busy and I already felt overwhelmed. I hoped the celestial RN spirits would listen and have pity.

I was reviewing orders for a patient I'll call "Jose." Jose had multiple gunshot wounds from gang-related street violence. He had a boyish face and a softhearted disposition, which was a visually confusing contradiction to the numerous symbol and name tattoos that appeared like a tired veil over his face, neck and chest. There were two packed wounds on his upper left chest where bullets rattled his trunk, as well as fresh wounds from removed bilateral chest tubes. Another bullet had penetrated through his left middle finger as he instinctively clutched the area of the initial gunshot wounds. The finger was amputated, his hand wrapped in a gauze dressing and his arm in a sling.

During the shift, Jose experienced multiple episodes of bilious emesis. He was in significant pain, yet continued to act quite stoic. Jose was also visibly weakened, his stomach revolting against the continued traumatic upset of his delicate internal balance. I had paged the doctor a few minutes earlier and was awaiting new orders to address his condition. Somewhere in my mind I was still hoping I could bypass any of those anxiety-laden skills for the rest of the day. I was so behind in my work, but I was also genuinely concerned for Jose – he was my priority.

I hit the refresh button on the computer screen to update the new orders, and there it was. My heart sank as the anticipation immediately started to build. It was as though each word delivered its own degree of anxiety. I read the order slowly, word by word. *Insert!* Oh no, I thought, nothing within my comfort zone is going to come from an order starting with "insert." *Insert Nasogastric Tube!* The nursing gods stood me up!

The rest of the order faded behind the main task. *125mmHg continuous suction* certainly was secondary information at that point. I quickly gathered my mental bearings. I knew I had to perform this task as soon as possible so my patient could feel relief from his heaving stomach. I knew my anxiety over inexperience needed to be a distant second to Jose's needs, although the internal conflict was taxing.

I did a quick review of NG tube insertion. One nurse told me to soak the tube in warm water so it would be more pliable. Another said to soak the tube in ice water so it's soothing to the throat. Conflicting advice from seasoned nurses is commonplace for the new nurse, and initially quite confusing. I decided to go with the method my preceptor practices instead of doing the "Sandy told me to..." or "that's not what Tim said" routine. I repeated the mantra "nose to earlobe to xiphoid process, nose to earlobe to xiphoid process" as I gathered the supplies.

I walked into the room and Jose looked as though he was gripped by affliction, his jaw repeatedly lunging forward and his tongue expelling from his mouth as he heaved bile into the pale rose-colored plastic basin. I was renewed in my purpose and my earlier prayers to the deaf nursing gods felt selfish. I still had some anxiety, but I felt committed to Jose as his nurse. The mounting pressure from the numerous incomplete tasks on my mental checklist became momentarily insignificant as well.

With my preceptor at my side, we informed Jose of the procedure, sat him in a high Fowler's position and set up the supplies. The clear NG tubing looked so large compared to his nostrils. I couldn't help but think that this was going to be an unpleasant experience for all involved. I measured the tubing and marked it with tape. We had previously medicated Jose with anti-emetics in a futile attempt to calm the retching that would likely be intensified with the insertion of plastic tubing down his esophagus. After choosing the best nare for insertion, I took a deep breath and started inserting the lubricated tube, attempting to direct it appropriately – although I didn't know exactly what that was or felt like.

Jose winced and tensed his facial muscles, reacting to the unnatural and painful stimulus. I tried to continue, inserting the tube as best I could. With the tube now likely in his pharynx, I instructed Jose to swallow and continue swallowing. Jose began to repeatedly and almost violently gag, I paused while he took a breath and I hesitated to continue. I knew my preceptor was intently observing my wavering hand. "Keep going," my preceptor softly whispered behind me. "You have to keep going."

At this point I started to lose what little confidence I had as I became more disturbed by his discomfort. I continued to advance the tubing despite my timorous thoughts. I could only meekly utter "swallow Jose, keep swallowing." I spotted tears on Jose's cheek, rolling over the inked tear drops underneath the corner of his eye. I looked down for a moment to steady my dominant hand when I noticed a drop of blood spatter into the basin resting on Jose's abdomen. I quickly looked back up at his face and the tip of his nose already had another drop of blood accumulating. That drop also spattered into the basin. At that exact moment, I spotted the tip of the NG tubing coming back out of his mouth as he continued to gag repeatedly, making passage into the esophagus difficult.

The view of the tubing coming back out of his mouth startled me as if it were some sort of a feral snake viciously popping out from an inconspicuous hole. I held my breath and again paused not knowing what to do. The trauma in his nostril continued to produce drops of blood falling into the basin of bile. I felt like I was failing at this. I didn't want to inflict anymore pain on Jose. I wanted to stop!

My hands began to sweat profusely in the blue nitrile gloves. My preceptor attempted to guide me through my next maneuver, but I slowly took a near invisible step backward signaling I needed her to take over. My preceptor took the tubing and slightly withdrew it from Jose's nostril, and in the same movement, she tactically manipulated the tubing while advancing it further.

Now a spectator, I put a hand on his shoulder, standing present in his pain. I attempted to encourage his fortitude and let him know I was still there for him. "You're doing great Jose. Almost there!" Within a few moments, the tubing appeared to be in the target place of his stomach and I continued encouraging and applauding him for his tolerance and bravery. Placement of the tubing was confirmed, and soon the bilious content that was plaguing his bloated abdomen quickly travelled (via 125mmHg of continuous suction) to the clear cylinder on the wall. I was relieved that Jose was okay, but during the rest of the shift, I carried around a distracting amount of disappointment and failure which took quite some time to fade.

Jose was on the unit a few more weeks, and was my patient several times. He continued to improve, and I enjoyed sharing in his recovery and celebrating his progress. I also witnessed him cope with the difficult fall from a previously invincible street ego to a young man dependent on others, needing his diaper changed, still overtaken by weakness and the unpredictability of a sick body. Eventually he continued to improve and was discharged, but he remained a patient whose situation and needs taught me a lot about myself, nursing, society and our interconnectedness.

One day a couple of months later, I was working on a different med/surg unit when the secretary told me someone was waiting at the desk to speak with me. I assumed it was a family member of a patient and walked over to the desk. I spotted a young man in baggy street clothes. When I was within a few steps from him, he said: "Well, I just wanted to say thank you."

I was caught off-guard and scanned my mind trying to recall which patient this young man could be associated with, and why he would be thanking me. Then I suddenly recognized the boyish face, gentle disposition and fading tattoos. It was Jose! His face had filled out and his skin color had regained a healthy glow. I was so surprised that I inadvertently dismissed his thanks and exclaimed, "Jose! You look great! I'm so happy for you!"

In his sheepish manner, he just repeated his words of gratitude, "Yeah well, I just wanted to thank you for everything." Then he walked away, not needing my acceptance, approval or conversation. As he continued to walk down the hall, I stood there with some lingering disbelief and a warm heart.

After finishing nursing school and starting a job, I had many conversations with fellow new nurses regarding skills (or lack thereof), how inept we felt and the plaguing inexperience that felt like an embarrassing disease. There was such a heavy emphasis on those anxiety-provoking tasks, which I felt throughout my orientation. I couldn't wait to feel comfortable, confident and competent so I could finally become, in my mind, a real nurse. When Jose came back to thank me, I realized he remembered much more than my traumatic NG tube insertion attempt or else he would never want to see my torturous hands again.

Patients like Jose feel compassion, presence and empathy and usually remember these in their time of great need. The acquisition of skills, recollection of policies and knowledge of procedures will come with exposure and experience, but if a genuine commitment of care, respect, compassion and presence is made to the patient, you can and will be a wonderful nurse on day one!

Laura Giambattista, BSN, RN, CMSRN
Graduated 2010

Your patients and families will always remember how you made them feel!

Our Preceptors and Mentors

"*The really great make you feel that you, too, can become great!*"

Mark Twain

The Blessing of My Preceptor

One of the richest blessings in my nursing career has been Maureen, my first preceptor as a new graduate nurse in pediatrics. While she honed and focused my nursing skills during that first year, the things she taught me about building therapeutic relationships with patients and families, collaborating with physicians and developing strong colleague relationships became the foundation of my nursing practice.

An early lesson I learned from Maureen was that a smile and a quiet voice go a long way. Even while feeling inner turmoil as a new grad, I needed to present a friendly, open posture and listen intently. In the midst of crying babies, anxious parents and rapid admissions, Maureen stayed calm and positive. When admitting a new patient, she didn't try to talk over the noise, but instead moved close to the parents – focusing on their concerns and outlining a brief plan so they knew what to expect. She created an atmosphere of trust through listening, acknowledging concerns and staying patient-centered.

Maureen was a master at collaborating with physician colleagues. I can still hear her voice ringing in my ear: "make a list of questions/concerns *BEFORE* you call the doctor, focus on what's most important first, have all the patient information in front of you and make suggestions about what the patient needs."

Maureen built an excellent reputation with physicians because she was organized, thorough with her assessment data and communicated clearly. When physicians entered the unit, she made a point of greeting them by name, asking who they wanted to see and locating the nurse to facilitate rounds. Even if she was in the middle of something, Maureen still took a moment to make a connection and build rapport.

She also created strong team relationships with her colleagues. Maureen often assisted with an admission without being asked, and would offer help to her colleagues prior to sitting down to chart. As we worked together, she taught me to have situational awareness regarding the atmosphere on the unit by noticing when a colleague was having a bad day, and providing encouragement and offering to help.

Maureen inspired me to finish each day with a question to myself: *What could I have done better today to improve my nursing care?* This is an excellent reflective question I've thought about as I've headed home from nursing shifts for more than 20 years. It represents the essence of Maureen's nursing practice and is the cornerstone of my own practice that she helped build.

Debra Brady, DNP, RN, CNS
Graduated 1989

Ask yourself: What can I do better to improve the care of my patients?

Nothing is as Bad as It Seems

The most valuable advice I received during my RN residency program was from my fabulous preceptor. I still remember her words: *Nothing is as bad as it seems!* It sounds simple, but this advice helps me keep things in perspective.

About halfway through my RN residency, I was coming on shift and noticed I was scheduled to care for a child with a myriad of metabolic and neurological issues. This baby was seriously ill. The mom was very involved in her child's care and had a reputation of being "difficult" and "needy." This family was often the talk of the break room before and after shifts. Just the night before, the mom had called a rapid response and the child was sent to the PICU. Lo and behold, they were back on my unit the next day. When I saw their name on my assignment, I immediately became tachycardic.

After a long dramatic report from the very stressed off-going nurse, I felt like I might need to grab an emesis basin. I turned to my very calm preceptor and said, "Okay, now I'm nervous about taking care of this kid!"

She replied, "If I can teach you anything during your residency it's this: nothing is as bad as it seems! Now let's assess the situation and make our own plan of care. It's all about communicating with the family and the patient. Remember that families are very stressed because their children are sick. We need to keep that in mind and be there for the family as well as the patient."

I looked at my preceptor and breathed a sigh of relief. She was right. I needed to make up my own mind and not assume the experience is going to be bad.

I went into the room and was pleasantly surprised when the mom turned out to be very helpful and thankful to us for the care we provided. The family had been through a lot, and by just anticipating their needs, the shift went smoothly.

I learned that by making my own decision to be open-minded and positive, my shift turned out to be a great learning experience.

Remember, *nothing is as bad as it seems!* Always take the opportunity to create the best experience for you, your patients and their families.

Kelly Navarro, RN, CPN
Graduated 2010

Don't let another team member's bad day influence you. Be open-minded and positive.

Finding Your Lifeline

When I graduated from nursing school with my BSN I was very comfortable with the theoretical aspects of my job. I'm a pretty organized person, so getting things done on schedule wasn't a problem either. My struggles revolved around confidence and comfort when completing treatments and procedures.

My first job was on a general medical/surgical floor of a teaching hospital. Patients ranged from pre-op cardiothoracic surgery, post-op cardiac catheterization, end-stage cancer and chemotherapy, to the chronically ill with a wide variety of diagnoses. Average age of our patients was around 80, and the length of stay for the chronically ill ranged from several days to months.

The nursing team dynamics were tense with many cliques and a young, inexperienced manager as our leader. I didn't know it until some time later, but because of my strong academic record, the manager told the staff that I was an up-and-coming star and they could learn a few things from me. The end result for me as a new team member was isolation and very little offers of help. I needed support!

The importance of having a BSN and an identity of professionalism were the underpinnings of my nursing program. I would have never imagined that my mentor and coach would be an LVN. Rosemary and I both started on the floor at the same time. She was an experienced LVN and had practiced in a small hospital ICU for several years. Life changes had brought her to this hospital which did not employ LVNs in critical care.

Rosemary became my lifeline! She was amazing in her ability to organize her day, and always seemed available to be with me when I had to do a procedure for the first time. She coached me through my first IV starts, catheterizations, wound irrigations and packing, and taught me the fine art of lung, bowel and heart auscultation.

When I look back at my first year of nursing, I know I wouldn't have survived without Rosemary. She held me up, pumped me full of confidence and with her as a mirror, I developed a can-do attitude.

It is so important to find people to support you as you begin your career. No matter what the dynamics are within the staff, you can succeed if you don't get sucked into those games, and instead focus on becoming the best nurse possible for your patients. In the end, my co-workers came to respect my diligence and even my ability to apply the theoretical foundations of my education to care dilemmas.

Although I was a strong believer in the value of having a degree, because of my initial difficulties on the floor, Rosemary thought I was proof that spending so much time in the classroom wasn't an asset for a bedside nurse. We had many friendly debates about this issue. Over the next several years our conversations changed as she obtained her associate degree in nursing and then progressed to BSN and then to MSN.

I love hearing her exclaim, "I had no idea how much I didn't know!" She is now a nurse executive in the same small hospital where she started as an LVN in the ICU.

Kay Evans, BSN, MAOL, RN
Graduated 1982

You can learn from all members of the health care team. Be open to what they can teach you.

Building Your Competence While Growing Your Confidence

As a new graduate nurse employed in the critical care unit of a large trauma center, I was very concerned about the vast amount of information that I believed I was expected to know. I thought I was supposed to know everything about critical care on the first day of work. Needless to say, this outlook caused me much anxiety.

One day during orientation, my preceptor called in sick and I was instructed to precept with Sherry, one of our seasoned nurses. Sherry had been a nurse for several decades and proudly shared that she recently achieved her national certification in critical care nursing (CCRN). To start our conversation, I asked Sherry what she thought about the CCRN examination. She said there was a heavy emphasis on neurology and she was glad she only had to take the exam once.

During that single night of orientation with Sherry, she taught me the most important lesson I still carry with me today. This is the same lesson I provide each of our new grad nurses to increase their competency and confidence in their knowledge base. Sherry instructed me to choose two medical diagnoses, preferably of the patients I was assigned to care for that evening, and read about these diagnoses when I was back home after the shift ended.

She suggested that I make this a habit every day I work in the unit. Since I worked three times a week, we calculated that by the end of 12 weeks I would have learned about 72 diagnoses. She reassured me that I would become more confident about my knowledge in three months. I felt the change in me within three weeks.

Every time I read about a medical diagnosis, I integrated the corresponding nursing diagnosis. I recalled patients and their family members. I remembered how they reacted not only to the diagnosis, but also to their entire hospital experience. Adding the emotional component of the experience enhanced my retention of the materials.

Knowledge is power! As I felt my knowledge grow, I became more confident in myself and was able to project that confidence in my daily assignments and interactions with patients and their loved ones. I encourage you to increase your confidence by developing effective reading habits.

Lourdes C. Salandanan, PhD(c), MSN, RN-BC, FNP
Graduated 1997

Expanding your knowledge base will increase your confidence and competence throughout your career.

234 Surviving and Thriving

Was It Early Just Culture?

Thinking back over my 43-year nursing career, many memories relate to my journey as an educator. However, there is one event that is as vivid as if it happened yesterday – my first significant error that may have contributed to a patient's death.

I say "may have" contributed rather than caused because the patient was unstable and receiving an anti-arrhythmic infusion to control an irritable cardiac rhythm. Let me set the stage...as a recent graduate with about three months experience in post-anesthesia recovery, I was hired into a relatively new acute care center that included ICU, CCU and NICU (as in neonatal ICU). Being clinically competent in all of those areas is another discussion for another day. The unit was a big square with nursing stations in the center, and all four sides of the unit visible from a nursing station. I worked the 3-11 shift, and this particular evening I was assigned to the CCU side.

My patient was a man in his 60s on an anti-arrhythmic drip to control premature ventricular contractions (PVCs). I provided care, comfort, patient teaching, counted the drops per minute (remember 43 years ago we didn't have IV pumps), watched the monitor and documented his cardiac rhythm, including his PVCs. I had studied EKGs, and knew that it was significant if there were more than six PVCs per minute. It had been a quiet shift, and I gave report and went home.

The next afternoon when I came to work, the charge nurse asked to see me. *Gasp! What had I done?* In a very professional, calm manner she showed me the EKG strip from the patient I had cared for the previous night – the strip I had placed in the chart. In just six inches of EKG paper there were three abnormal looking beats in a row – not six in a minute, but a run of V-tach. The patient had arrested and died during the night shift.

I documented the rhythm, but had not intervened for the V-tach. *Why?* Because I didn't know a run of PVCs was V-tach or that it was any more significant than six PVCs in a minute. I can still see my manager's face when she told me the patient had arrested! Did I even assess the patient for a change? Did I just mount the strip in the chart? I didn't give the IV bolus of Lidocaine that was ordered for such episodes.

I believe I experienced the *Just Culture* philosophy before there was such a system in healthcare. My manager used the opportunity to review my mistake, discuss additional education that would enhance my practice in the CCU, and she supported *ME*, who was in tears.

Just Culture says "we must coach our employees to be consistent and honest in their behaviors, help them make the best choices and learn from their mistakes." To be a nurse is to be a lifelong learner. Studying didn't end when I graduated…it had just begun.

As a new graduate I was eager, passionate, inexperienced and vulnerable. I received the support I needed. I was consoled by my manager, but I was also accountable for my actions. Throughout my career, I have consistently focused on achieving the best possible outcomes for my patients (and my students!).

During my nursing education, our fundamentals faculty member handed us a piece of paper with the following quote: *The road is rough, but you can make it. Hold out your hand and God will take it.*

I pasted that quote in my pocket resource book, and have repeated it to myself time and time again. In addition to your belief system, do not hesitate to reach out as a new graduate – you are not alone in your professional journey. Thanks for choosing nursing as your career!

Robyn Nelson, PhD, RN
Graduated 1970

At times, the road may be rough, but the journey is worth it!

What Would Florence Do?

I remember my orientation as a new graduate nurse as if it were yesterday. It was a hot week in August, and the orientation classroom's air conditioning was not working. There were more than 20 new graduate RNs in the class with me. I had no idea that our orientation was going to be all about lectures and testing.

"Not dosage calculations again!" I almost screamed. Nursing school was tough enough, but it was well worth it now that I had my license. After two days of classroom activities and testing, I passed the dosage calculation exam. That meant I was able to proceed to hospital orientation.

Even though the first semester of nursing school was scary, it was nothing like my first month in the hospital as a novice graduate nurse. I was scared to death, but confident in my theoretical knowledge. I was hired to the obstetric unit and was scheduled for 3½ weeks of orientation there.

I really had no idea what was in store for me as I began my orientation on the unit. It was very busy. There were days when I went home crying because I was tired and frustrated from the long 12-hour shifts and the lack of a consistent support system. Because my assigned preceptor was always very busy, my source of peace became the words of nursing theorists and what I had learned in nursing school about how to manage and cope with illness and stress.

The blending of theory and practice in nursing is called praxis. It may sound surprising to new nurses, but I love nursing theory. There are some praxis theorists I still look to today to get me and my patients or co-workers through a busy day at work or at the hospital.

Three nursing theorists who are especially important to me are Jean Watson, Patricia Benner and Florence Nightingale. Watson's caring theory, Benner's novice to expert model and Nightingale's passion for nursing have helped me get through many difficult situations.

These theorists are a permanent and consistent lifeline to help me in times of crisis. I definitely utilized their wisdom during my orientation as a new graduate.

I will never forget walking into Jenny's dark room one night during my hospital orientation. Jenny was pregnant and suffering from preeclampsia. An intern had discontinued her magnesium sulfate infusion and then left the unit to take a nap. For the past two days, Jenny's blood pressure had been controlled with this medication. Based on one critical lab result on Jenny's chart, the intern had stopped her mag sulfate without rechecking her lab work. Her last recorded BP while on mag sulfate was 110/72.

I was monitoring Jenny closely. At 2 a.m., nearly three hours after her mag sulfate infusion was stopped, her supine blood pressure was 160/98, the same BP she had when admitted to the hospital. I asked Jenny to sit up so I could take her BP again. This time it rose to 178/104. Her face was puffy and she was having trouble seeing the images on the television. "I can't see the picture on the screen," Jenny said. I told her I was going to call her doctor and immediately left the room.

I made three attempts to contact the intern before he returned my call. Instead of coming down to examine Jenny, he asked me to take her BP again and draw some lab work to check her electrolytes. I asked if we should restart the mag sulfate after drawing the blood, but he said, "No, let's wait for the lab results." After drawing the blood and rechecking the blood pressure (which was still high), I became very worried and consulted with my assigned preceptor, who was still very busy with her laboring patient.

I remembered the nursing theorists who are so important to me. What would they do in this situation? Gaining strength from their dedication to patient care, I insisted that my preceptor call the intern or resident to come and evaluate Jenny. I could not allow the intern to continue to sleep while my patient and her baby were at risk.

Due to this intervention and insistence that the physician check on his patient, Jenny and her premature baby came through with no complications following an emergency cesarean section.

As nurses we work in caring/healing environments on a daily basis. Nursing gives us the ability to help change society through our education, actions and beliefs that all persons are equal and have the same human origins.

The moment Jenny said thank you to me before being discharged, I knew I would never forget her or that caring praxis moment. This experience reminds me of the benefits of utilizing the wisdom of nursing theorists. Socialization and understanding of nursing theories can help novice nurses advance to competency and beyond.

Mercy Popoola, PhD, RN, CNS
Graduated 1984

The art of nursing involves the successful blending of theory and practice.

Even New Grads Can Take Charge

Time management will make or break you. This is where a good preceptor can make all the difference.

I was hired onto a unit where I had worked as a nursing assistant while going to nursing school. I was grateful to have the position and considered myself lucky to be in a place where I already knew the layout and the staff. The manager invited my input for my preceptor and I suggested Laura, a seasoned RN who liked to teach, had a relaxed air about her and had a background similar to mine – a mom of school-aged kids and a second career in nursing.

What I didn't realize is that nursing school fills your head with the *what* and *why* of caring for patients, but it cannot prepare you for the *how* of managing a patient assignment. That happens on the job as you gain experience.

Laura started me out with a one-patient assignment, reviewing my skill competencies and necessary documentation. Over the next three weeks, I progressed to caring for 3-4 patients, a typical assignment for our high-acuity unit. As I worked, Laura would talk about the underlying disease process, the pharmokinetics of certain drugs or other interesting and useful topics. When I was faced with multiple tasks all due at the same time, Laura would talk me through the prioritization and then cheerfully go off and take care of a task or two to "catch me up."

Sounds great, right? *Wrong!* What I didn't understand or identify until later was that by Laura talking at me most of the time (instead of with me), my brain was full of her thoughts. I wasn't really doing my own thinking/problem solving/time management. I wasn't moving towards the independence I needed in order to be safe.

At the fourth week, Laura wanted me to do as much of the assignment as possible without her help, so she stepped aside. But on this day, I found myself immediately facing a perfect storm of new nursing tasks and decisions I simply did not know how to execute.

Here's what was happening:

- I had a patient who was NPO and had been given his 0600 sliding scale and basal insulin doses. *Will he become hypoglycemic? How often should I recheck his glucose level? Do I need to inform the MD?*

- A patient is scheduled for 0800 dialysis. *Do I call someone for this? What about morning meds? Breakfast?*

- I received a critical lab value and the resident covering the patient had not yet turned on his pager. *Now who do I call? Do we give blood before dialysis? What do I do about high calcium?*

- I was paged because my non-English speaking patient complained of chest pain. *What are the standard cardiac orders? When do we break out the crash cart? And wait a minute – she was supposed to be my "stable" patient!*

Later, this patient's troponin levels came back elevated and orders were written for a transfer to a monitored bed. *How does a unit transfer happen? What does the RN do? You mean I'm supposed to travel with her? But I'm not ACLS certified!*

- By now patient #1's IV antibiotic was late and it was not in his bin. *The satellite pharmacy's door was closed. How do I get a medication from the central pharmacy?*

My uncertainty seemed endless and I felt defeated. Laura came to my rescue, cheerfully talking all the time about what was happening as we worked through that morning's chaos. But even though she was willing to patiently teach me what I needed to know, my head was "overfull." I couldn't hear a thing she was saying!

I needed to approach my transition differently. I was going to be on my own soon and felt I had way too many "I don't know how" questions. I spoke with the manager. We decided to change preceptors and my manager chose a nurse not very far out of nursing school herself – just a year ahead of me.

What a change! My new preceptor didn't talk much. Instead she let me think, let me tell her my plan, had me ask for help only when I really needed it, and even then, coached me instead of taking over. Her focus was much more centered on accomplishing the needed tasks. There were often questions she couldn't answer about the diseases or treatments. When that happened, her response was always, "good question – let's look it up" or "let's ask someone who has been here longer."

She patterned for me how to problem-solve in the context of our unit, where to find reliable resources and how to get the charting and tasks done on time. In hindsight, each preceptor taught me different, but equally valuable skills. I'm grateful to both of them for their patience and faith as I worked to become safe and competent on the floor.

So what is my advice to new grads? Speak up for yourself when things aren't working. Time management will make or break you. I was reluctant to tell my manager that I wasn't learning what I needed from the preceptor I had requested. I feared that somehow she would think I wasn't capable of becoming independent and question hiring me.

But in taking the risk and talking with my manager, I ended up with a much better learning situation for me and became a stronger new nurse for my patients.

Jennifer M. Friedenbach, MSN, RN, CNL, CMSRN
Graduated 2008

Speak up to seek the learning experiences you need to grow.

The Health Care Team:
Together We're Stronger!

"Alone we can do little. Together we can do much!"

The Nerve Center

Of all the insights I've had into nursing during my first year, the greatest was my realization that the RN is a nerve center, the main link between the patient and everyone else.

One day I was caring for a 47 year-old woman from rural Mexico. She had a history of wildly uncontrolled diabetes and was admitted with osteomyelitis of a toe, which was then amputated. She spoke no English and was illiterate. She had never taken insulin, but the MD wanted to start her on both long-acting and sliding-scale coverage before meals and at bedtime. She was scheduled for discharge later that day and one of my orders was to provide diabetes education. She was unable to walk more than a few feet, had vomited recently and was still nauseous despite receiving antiemetic medications.

Here's a list of some of the people I spoke with, many of them extensively: doctors from both services managing her care, the patient and her extended family, the pharmacist, the financial services representative, our unit secretary, our nursing assistants, the nutritionist, the physical therapist, the occupational therapist and other experienced RNs for consultation. The most important thing I accomplished was working with the physicians to nix the idea of sliding-scale insulin coverage. But there were also many other challenges we overcame in order to safely discharge this patient.

Consider what might have happened without the nurse: the patient would have received a dangerously complex insulin prescription (being that she was illiterate and unable to draw up the correct amount of insulin, let alone interpret a sliding-scale); she may have left the hospital before she was well enough; she wouldn't be able to fill her prescriptions because she couldn't afford them; she also might not have received her walker, dietary advice or the emphasis on the importance of future follow-up for her diabetes.

I don't say all of this to toot my own horn. Actually, I would have been ineffective in this situation without the tremendous help I got from everyone else. The revelation I had was just how much the nurse's job consists of nearly constant communication with so many team members.

Chris Poole, BSN, RN
Graduated 2010

Nursing is the glue binding the health care team!

The Art of Listening

Our first jobs as registered nurses are often both thrilling and frightening! Within weeks of graduating from my nursing program, I discovered I had a great deal more to learn and that I was just darn lucky in this situation. My self-confidence about my strong listening skills may have been a bit unwarranted.

I chose to attend a three-year nursing diploma program because of its reputation in producing outstanding clinical nurses. During our last year of training, we nursing students had the opportunity to be team leaders on busy nursing units, with nursing students on all three shifts and experienced RNs to provide support and mentoring.

When I graduated, I felt very confident in accepting a position at that same hospital as a team leader on the evening shift of a 48-bed medical/surgical unit. I chose the 3-11 p.m. shift because I liked to work later in the day – having my mornings off and the ability to go out after work with my friends. An added benefit in my young eyes was that all those "administrative types" were off duty by then and weren't there to hassle us or be looking over our shoulders. I also felt that I would have the opportunity to learn and settle into my RN role more quickly through what I considered to be a more independent practice.

The RN I worked with most frequently was very experienced and provided excellent support and guidance. On one particular occasion during my first few weeks, I quickly learned the importance of listening to members of my team and the value of assessing patients personally.

On the unit, there were two RN team leaders working with nursing assistants and LPNs (LVNs) along with one or two additional RNs. One evening I was preparing patient medications in the med room.

At that time, we didn't have many single dose medications. We actually used little 1x1 inch cards for each separate medication along with a med tray with small cups for each patient's meds.

We'd been at work for a few hours when one of the experienced nursing assistants on my team told me that one of the patients she was assigned to feed didn't want to eat. Since I was focused on prepaing the medications and didn't want to be distracted, I told her to go back to the patient's room and work with the patient to get him to eat at least a little. I was aware the patient was on a soft diet, so I knew it shouldn't be too difficult for him to eat the food on his tray. The nursing assistant came back shortly and said she wasn't able to convince him to eat. I told her to keep trying, then left the room with my full med tray to start passing medications to my patients.

After I had been to a couple rooms, the nursing assistant came back and told me that the patient still refused to eat. I told her I would go see him right away and led the way to the patient's room. He was sitting straight up in bed, but unfortunately I discovered he wasn't breathing! Since I knew he was a "DNR" I checked and found no pulse either.

I sent the nursing assistant to get the other RN team leader. We contacted the physician who was in the hospital. As we were waiting for the physician to arrive in order to pronounce the patient, I closed the patient's eyes and I noticed something on his lip. Imagine my surprise when I checked further and discovered that his mouth was still completely full of mashed potatoes!

That night I learned that I needed to listen, really listen, to members of my team and to "hear" what they were telling me. I realized that I should be asking questions and even more importantly, when experienced staff members are telling me information repeatedly, I need to follow-through and personally assess the patient myself.

To this day anytime I see a "DNR" order, I also have a vivid picture of that expired patient sitting straight up in bed with his mouth filled with mashed potatoes!

Peggy Diller, MS, RN, NE-BC
2006 ACNL President
Graduated 1969

Two key steps in delegation are listening and following-up.

Staying Positive Through Adversity

I was in my first year of graduate school and needed a part-time job to support myself while in school. I accepted a position in the ICU of a renowned teaching hospital. I was very excited about what I would learn in a busy ICU. My previous ICU experience had been at a community hospital in my hometown in Massachusetts.

Everything went well during my orientation. I was then assigned to work evenings, which was the shift I requested. However on several occasions, I was left alone to admit a fresh open-heart surgery patient, to care for a severely infected MRSA patient or to take care of patients who had been on the unit for extended lengths of stay.

When I shared my concern that I needed more support to transition into this new position, the response was: "You're in graduate school. Since you're so smart, you should be able to figure out what to do. You're on your own!"

At first I was put-off by these remarks. Then I decided to take it in stride, to give the best care I could, and do it with a good attitude and a smile. I rarely talked about what I was learning in graduate school, and I found not sharinig this new knowledge to be very frustrating. But I must have done something right, because when I left the cardiac surgical ICU, the staff on my shift had a special celebration for me. It was one of the best going away parties I've had in my career!

My caring attitude and ability to get the job done was what mattered most in the end. This experience taught me to persevere for my patient's well-being, no matter how difficult the work environment may be.

I have made it a priority since that time to encourage healthy work environments and to make sure new grads or new hire nurses get what they need to be successful. I don't want others to feel the way I was made to feel so many years ago. It was truly a turning point in my professional life.

Suzette Cardin, DNSc, RN, FAAN
Graduated 1970

Maintaining a positive attitude, demonstrating competence and remaining focused on our patients can overcome conflict and adversity.

Better Care Through Effective Teams

It was 1974, and I was so lucky to be hired into one of the RN roles at the hospital where I had completed several of my clinical rotations. This hospital was in the inner city of Queens, New York. It was a poor, dangerous community with high crime rates and a newly funded methadone clinic that supported over 450 heroin addicts.

Besides typical medical/surgical diagnoses, our patients were hospitalized for stabbings, gunshot wounds, drug overdoses, pelvic inflammatory diseases from chronic prostitution, as well as other injuries or illnesses related to violence and poverty. Many of our patients were addicted to drugs.

The med/surg unit was 30 beds with two large 12-bed wards on each end. I worked variable shifts as well as the eight-hour day shift. We had a team-based model in which I typically cared for 15 patients with one LVN, who helped with medications and treatments, and one nursing assistant. When I worked the night shift, I was the only nurse caring for 30 patients with one nursing assistant, usually Bessie, Emma or Ernie.

My fellow team members taught me so much! I learned direction, organization, delegation and communication skills from Ms. G, our head nurse. Ms. G taught me to be an effective team leader by balancing clear and direct communication with strong listening skills. Through her example, I learned to lead our team with respect and professionalism. She was also thoughtful, firm and respectfully directive with the medical interns and residents – quite a valuable talent.

Bessie, Emma and Ernie, our nursing assistants, taught me some of the most worthwhile lessons about being an effective team player. They were expert at so many techniques I didn't know about as a new nurse.

I learned to do exceptional, caring and efficient baths and dressing changes. I marveled at their ability to conduct culturally competent, thoughtful, therapeutic and nonjudgmental conversations with our patients. These patients were tough as nails from living on the streets of this poor, ravaged community, yet they were so frightened of being hospitalized. Through their caring and compassion, Bessie, Emma and Ernie helped put these patients at ease to aid the healing process.

These three nursing assistants also modeled the importance of treating each and every team member with respect and caring to foster team synergy. Finally, they taught me to effectively manage conflict. They never avoided conflict, but instead used a direct approach to resolve the issue and move on to more important matters.

I am grateful for these early influencers in my nursing career – they helped shape my skills as a team member. Since that first job, I've learned innumerable lessons from other team members along the way.

There is so much to learn in nursing and so many opportunities to grow. This is why we must be committed to learning from each other and sharing our knowledge with other members of the health care team, no matter what their role.

Kathy Harren, MSN, MHS, RN, NEA-BC
2007 ACNL President
Graduated 1974

Respect, trust and excellent communication skills are key components of effective teams.

Message on My Lunch Bag

As a nurse with one year of experience under my belt, I moved to a rural community and started a new job as a labor and delivery nurse. I was extremely nervous my first day of work, since I knew very little about birthing babies, and I had heard stories of the "war-horse" nurse manager who would be overseeing my training.

I spent the morning trying to make the best impression possible and by lunchtime, she was starting to warm up to me. This was until I retrieved the lunch my husband had packed me from the refrigerator. Unbeknownst to me, my husband, who was my number one fan, had written on the lunch bag: "Kathy Cocking, Director of Nursing." I found it hysterical and endearing, but the nurse manager did not! The rest of my orientation was a very chilly affair.

This experience was a great learning on two fronts. First, it shaped the way I oriented new employees once I was in a position to act as a preceptor. I was able to empathize with their novice status, as well as their excitement and nervousness about a new job. I challenged myself to have a very positive influence on their orientation experience so that they would have a very different learning memory to share.

In addition, dealing with a manager I didn't see eye-to-eye with taught me fortitude and persistence. Although not all coworkers and bosses would be my best friends, I could work with them harmoniously by demonstrating competence, willingness to learn and professionalism.

And by the way, my husband must have had a premonition – within six years I was promoted to the director of nursing role!

Kathy Cocking, MSN, RN
Graduated 1978

Don't let obstacles get in the way of your success...

Taking Care of Each Other

Today I am a nursing instructor. As a new graduate nurse in 1988, I never thought my career path would be nursing education. Like most new grads, there was so much about nursing I didn't understand.

My first job was in the pediatric intensive care unit, scheduled for a month of days and a month of nights. It was a rough first year with all the flipping of shifts. Besides the stress, I was also sick several times. Pediatric nurses frequently get sick their first year – being around kids, I guess. After one particular night shift, I was exhausted! So tired, it was even difficult to fall asleep. I did my usual routine to relax for sleep, but it took me a couple of hours to really fall asleep.

And boy, did I sleep! For 14 hours!

Shocked, I woke up to a loud knock on my door. Who was there, but a police officer! Apparently, the PICU staff was so worried when I didn't show up for the night shift, that they phoned the police to check on me. I threw on my uniform and headed to work. I was so stressed on the drive to work. My mind was racing: *I'm going to get fired! Being sick, missing so many days of work and now this!*

When I ran in the door, the nurses hugged me, saying they were glad I was okay. I was so relieved. That is what nursing is all about. Taking care of our patients and of each other. And having more than one alarm clock to wake you up!

Bridget Parsh, EdD, MSN, RN, CNS
Graduated 1988

We do our best work caring for patients when we also care about each other.

Finding Your Path

"*Destiny is not a matter of chance, it is a matter of choice. It is not a thing to be waited for, it is a thing to be achieved.*"

William Jennings Bryan

The Sweetest Profession of All

My previous career revolved around desserts: inventing them, baking them and taste testing them. It was a delicious job and upon learning about what I did, people would respond with: "Mmmmm . . . you're so lucky!"

And it truly was fun – eating warm, flaky croissants for lunch and whipping up mango mousse. But after a few years of working with sugar and butter, I couldn't help but think about the trivialness of my career. The biggest impact I was making in a person's life was the widening of their waistband.

I began taking classes at night. If I wanted a career that wasn't trivial, a career that could actually change a person's life, then I would have to take off my apron and get into some scrubs. Nursing seemed to offer all the things I was looking for. After two years of classes, including an accelerated nursing degree, I became an RN.

When I first considered leaving desserts for nursing, I thought I would feel that my new job was more worthwhile. But I had no idea how truly fulfilling nursing would be! Beyond being able to care for my patients' health, it is a privilege to share in people's lives. And I've learned how extraordinary a seemingly "normal" life is.

While I will always have a soft spot in my heart for desserts, I am forever happy that I changed careers. Caring for people is the best job there is – even sweeter than cakes and cookies!

Kendra Bartlow, BSN, RN, OCN
Graduated 2009

Nurses have the privilege of sharing in people's lives!

Nursing: It's My Calling

It's 8 p.m. on the adolescent unit of an urban hospital. Of the many tasks to be accomplished: a teenage cystic fibrosis patient is requesting a bedding change, Cisplatin needs to be reconstituted and the IV tubing for the drip must be foil wrapped, a commode is ready for pick up in central supply, parents require diabetic education and chest percussion therapy is needed for patients with respiratory problems.

This was a typical night for me as a new graduate nurse. However, this night was different from all others. I went into Room 22 to find a very weak and frail 17 year old cystic fibrosis (CF) patient who had been in the hospital most of my six months as a new nurse. Our hospital was a regional referral center for CF and we had many CF patients on the adolescent side. During the 70s and 80s, pediatric units were divided by age rather than diagnosis, as they are today. I was the only RN on the evening shift for the 22-bed adolescent unit, with one nursing assistant.

My very thin, frail CF patient asked me if I would change her sheets because she was sweating profusely and had soiled them. My nursing assistant was busy, so I grabbed the linens from the cart and came back to her room. My patient was alone and dozing in and out.

Her body was so weak, I was almost afraid to move her. I got the sheets under her on one side, and asked her to turn over so I could quickly do the other side. After getting the sheets neat and tidy, I turned her to face me. When I looked into her eyes, they were glazed and she was not breathing. It was as though she had fallen quietly asleep in my arms.

Over the past few weeks, I knew she was reaching the end of her life in her debilitated, fragile state. But I never thought it would happen like this – in my arms! I hugged her close to my body and started to cry, just as I am now writing about my first patient to die in my care.

I thought to myself, *How can I cry when there are so many other things to do and so many other patients to take care of?* But at that moment, I knew she needed me just as much as I needed to be with her. This ultimate state of peacefulness and calmness when being with someone as they take their last breath of life was something I had never experienced up to this point.

This very profound experience left a lasting impression on me personally and professionally. Personally, I felt I had a special gift to give to my patients, and later to my beloved family members. This gift is the art of comforting someone in their last moments of life.

On two subsequent occasions, I was alone with my grandmother and brother when the end was near and they died in my arms. I have been told I have a "special calling" to support and cope with death in its final moments. I attribute this trait to being a nurse. We support people at their most vulnerable moments, whether it is a painful procedure, a medication that will make them ill or holding them when they are dying.

I wanted to be a nurse since I was about six years old. In fact, I still have a copy of a composition I wrote in first grade about what I wanted to be when I grew up. The death of my first patient, as well as many other patient experiences since, inspired me to further my professional development beyond bedside nursing.

First, I thought I wanted to become a nurse practitioner so I could write orders for my patients instead of always following the physician's orders. I entered a part-time graduate nursing program which gave me the opportunity to attend school and continue to work.

The program was a master's in science with a major in nursing administration, with the option to continue on for an additional year to become a nurse practitioner. As I was finishing my MSN degree, I decided not to pursue the nurse practitioner option and instead continue my nursing career as an administrator. I believed that as a nurse administrator, I would have the sphere of control and influence to improve patient care on a large scale.

A few years ago, one of my dreams came true. Almost four years in the making, I was able to build a comprehensive pediatric cancer center. After the facility opened, I frequently rounded to talk with patients and families to find out what they thought of our new center. Their positive feedback gave me the heartfelt satisfaction I had envisioned. I realized that if you set a dream, then you often have the power and influence to make it happen. Reaching this goal has not caused me to stop pursuing my passion and dreams to make an even greater impact on as many patients' lives as I can. I will continue to strive even further in pursuing this personal challenge.

You might say it all started with the passing of my first patient within the first six months of my career. I must admit this experience had a tremendous impact on my life. Most significant was the realization of the fragility of not just that teenage patient, but of life itself.

I encourage you to live life to its fullest and make the greatest impact you can. You will find personal satisfaction and develop into a fulfilled professional who is answering their "calling" in life!

Susan Herman, DNP(c), MSN, RN
Graduated 1978

Make your dreams come true for yourself and your patients.

Beginning My Journey

This is a story about my journey as a new RN. I cherished becoming a nurse and being a nurse.

As a new grad, I was fortunate to secure employment that included a 16-week internship at a small community hospital. Although I was hired into the critical care unit, I was first assigned to work in the medical/surgical units. At that time, med/surg units were thought to provide new graduates with a realistic experience for organizing patient care. Being assigned 15-20 patients or more certainly created the necessity to become better organized. Looking back, I happily received my assignment and went gliding blissfully to care for my patients. Today, laws prohibit the very thought of organizing care for more than five patients.

As a new grad, my preceptor was my role model for professional practice. I carefully noted how she received report, wrote and kept her notes on the patients, communicated with the physicians, managed her time and prepared to hand-off her patients at the end of the shift.

I poured my energy into becoming a good nurse. My goal was to excel as a critical care nurse. There came a point when I needed to care for more complex patients in order to continue to grow.

I then transferred to a tertiary care center as my new graduate days came to a close. As time passed and my practice matured, my journey has taken many paths. To this day, I cherish my career as an RN and all the wonderful experiences and oppotunities nursing has provided.

Sandra K. Davis, PhD, RN
Graduated 1978

Don't be afraid to redefine your path in nursing.

When You Know, You Know

I had always heard that when working with children, you are not only treating the child, but a very stressed family as well. Children are often the happiness and source of energy for families. When one is hospitalized, it often throws the whole family out of balance. Parents become anxious and stressed about not being able to help their child, and their behavior is often interpreted as being "difficult."

I became a pediatric nurse because I wanted to take care of sick kids. And not just because I wanted to help them get better, but because their courage and hope is undeniably contagious. I know family-centered care is important, but as a new nurse I really just wanted to focus on my patients.

Not long after starting my RN residency, I found myself caring for a difficult family. It was a mother of a total care kid who was making my day extremely difficult. Everything I did had to be on the mother's time schedule and exactly the way she wanted.

Daily care and tasks ended up taking much more time than needed, and I found myself falling behind throughout the day. I kept thinking that this woman was just trying to make me work twice as hard so she could watch me struggle. I continued to do everything just the way she wanted, and by the end of the day I began to catch up with my duties and settle into a groove.

I left the hospital that day feeling completely unappreciated. I felt that I went above and beyond what was required of me as a nurse, but didn't feel like it made a difference to the patient or the mother. I went back the next day knowing that I was in for another long day, but I found that it wasn't so bad. I remembered how the mom liked things done, and realized it didn't really take that much longer to accommodate her needs. The day went on and I left not thinking twice about it.

A few weeks later I came to work, and in my mailbox was a *Paw Print*, our organization's form of recognition, along with a note from the "difficult" mother of my patient. In her note, she expressed gratitude for the compassion I showed her son during their stay, and how my actions helped her through this difficult time. I was so touched she had noticed and took the time to thank me. It made everything I did that day and everyday worthwhile.

Now I know that I became a nurse to help, not only my patients, but also the families impacted by a child's illness. Whenever I am having a long day with parents stressing me out, I think about this mother's note, and it makes it all worthwhile. Now I know this is what I am supposed to do in life and that I am making a difference.

Kendall Quick, BSN, RN, CPN
Graduated 2010

Behind every patient is their family – whether traditional or nontraditional.

The Question

The question is worded in many ways, but no matter the posture or structure, it essentially asks the same thing: *Isn't it difficult working with sick babies?*

My mother always says life is like a pendulum when it comes to emotions. The further the pendulum swings one way, the further it can swing the opposite way. Therefore, greater sadness innately allows for greater joy. My experience in the RN residency program at a children's hospital has solidified this concept in my mind and heart. So now, each time someone asks me *the question*, I explain to them the concept of this pendulum – that although there is the potential for great sadness, there is also the potential for great joy. And this is how I approach my job.

Being a new grad in the pediatric cardiovascular ICU has provided me with some incredible experiences, and I can't begin to imagine what the future has in store. I love my job caring for high acuity patients. Ultimately our goal as nurses is for healing, for saving lives and for enabling children to leave the hospital and live outside our world of medicine.

One day in particular stands out to me. I had a two-patient assignment, and both my young charges were relatively stable and most likely going home the next day. As an ICU nurse there is something inside of me that loves taking care of the really sick kids, which is probably why I chose the ICU. However, that day I got a glimpse of something precious!

One of my patients was a baby girl who was recovering from a double outlet right ventricle and ventricular septal defect surgical repair. Toward the end of the day when I was caught up with everything, I was able to take her off the monitor and bring her out to the nurses' station to feed her. After she finished her bottle, my preceptor and I just sat and played with her. While holding this beautiful baby – listening to her laugh, watching her take in her surroundings, singing songs to her and making funny faces with her – my pendulum swung all the way to joy.

Although this is not what the majority of my days are like, it was a great reminder of what we're working toward as nurses. For what greater joy is there than to see patients and their families through what might be the lowest and most vulnerable time in their lives, and be joy for them? This kind of joy isn't the same as happiness. It's not a perky, go-lucky attitude that says everything is going to be all right. Instead it's a constancy – a cheerfulness and contentedness that conveys the message: *You are cared for!*

It is for this reason that I am able to joyfully explain why I do what I do and when answering *the question.*

Allison Greene, BSN, RN, CCRN
Graduated 2010

Find joy in what you do…it will help you overcome the moments of sadness.

Forging New Paths

I graduated in the top 10 percent of my nursing class and was presented with my school's nursing student excellence award. Yet, I could not land a job after graduation. I began my employment search by trying to get my dream job in pediatrics, but quickly switched to seeking a nursing job in any area.

After a year, I was told I was an "old" new grad, and would not be considered for any of the new grad positions available. While attending a nursing event, I connected with a friend from nursing school who worked at an ambulance company doing critical care transports. With her recommendation, I landed my first nursing job at the ambulance company.

Prior to securing this position, I didn't even known that nurses worked on ambulances, so I didn't know what to expect from the job. However, I learned the importance of being open to new possibilities and being accepting of opportunities that come your way – even if it's not what you anticipated. I love nursing, and knew that as long as I could work as an RN, I would be happy.

As an RN on the ambulance, I was now transporting patients while providing interventions and performing a wide range of nursing skills (running a ventilator, IV pumps, etc.). During my first few months, I felt like I was out of my depth, especially since completing my orientation period. After orientation, it was just me with two EMTs (one of whom would be driving) on each transport.

To feel more confident, I completed five certification courses in my first three months. In addition, for many of the medical conditions I saw most often during my transports, I kept reference materials on hand to consult in case complications arose. I prepared for the worst by running scenarios in my mind so that if something happened I would act appropriately and not freeze up. Part of preparing for the worst was always having emergency supplies available during transit from the hospital room to the ambulance (ambu bag, oxygen, defibrillator, and any medications I might need to administer) just in case my patient began to crash in the elevator or hallway.

The best advice I can share with new nurses is to be confident in front of your patients. No matter how worried I felt, when patients believed I was in control of the situation, they usually remained calm and their vital signs were more stable – which helped to prevent complications from occurring in the first place.

Always use your resources and ask questions if you're unsure about what to do. For example, I was transporting a patient on a ventilator whose oxygen saturation dropped from the 90s to 80s in the ambulance. I changed settings, checked tubing and I still couldn't get their O_2 sat level higher. So I called a coworker for advice. The simple answer I received was to take the ventilator out of the equation and just use an ambu bag to provide oxygenation. The patient's oxygen saturation immediately came back to baseline and they were stable for the rest of the trip.

Machines are not always the answer and sometimes we must step back and remember we're treating the patient, not the equipment!

Carrie Garland, BSN, RN
Graduated 2008

Be open to possibilities – you never know what opportunity lies ahead.

My "Almost" First Nursing Job

This job was really not my first, but in many ways it felt like it! After graduation from nursing school, I worked in labor and delivery for several years and ultimately became a head nurse. Then I made the decision to stay at home to raise a family.

Eventually, I needed to go back to work to help support my family. Nursing practice changes constantly and it had been more than 10 years since I worked as an RN. I still remembered the basics, but was completely behind on anything current. So I enrolled in a nursing refresher course. Although I was filled with trepidation when starting the course, I found it very interesting studying the different aspects of nursing practice that were covered.

Armed with this new knowledge, I applied for a position at a local hospital. The nursing supervisor who interviewed me seemed a little uncertain about hiring me, but fortunately she did. Since this was a new and unknown experience, I elected to be a per diem employee as a "six to tenner," a staff nurse who worked 6-10 p.m. to augment the evening shift staff and help with HS and other care. It also meant floating to different units, so I quickly became familiar with the hospital.

In many ways it felt like being a new grad again because so much was different. Nurses had much more responsibility and autonomy and performed so many more procedures that I recalled physicians doing before. On the other hand, like getting back on a bicycle, so much came back to me that I quickly realized I still knew how to care for patients. My skills may have been rusty, but the nursing process remained. I will always be grateful to the nurses I worked with who were welcoming, supportive and helped me gain confidence. I went on to accept a position on the evening shift of the med/surg unit, and worked for several years with a fine group of nurses. I later moved into nursing management and then teaching.

I chose this med/surg unit because there were several experienced nurses who understood the importance of mentoring. It's essential for novice nurses to have role models and mentors, who not only practice safely and with compassion, but understand that new nurses haven't yet mastered all the competencies. They must be patient and help these new nurses learn and grow. Unfortunately some workplaces have nurses who aren't willing to help. Usually new RNs identify those folks early, and whenever possible, approach the nurses who will support them. It's important to look for those colleagues who are willing to help you be successful.

New nurses also have the responsibility to continue learning since graduation is just the start of their journey to excel. Taking classes beyond those that are mandatory, subscribing to journals and pursuing higher degrees are all important ways to show that you want to be the best nurse possible. Your nurse colleagues will recognize this.

One always hopes that all new nurses will have rewarding experiences. I was fortunate with my "almost" first job!

Alison Riggs, MSN, RN, ONC
Graduated 1956

As RNs, it's our responsibility to help new nurses learn and grow.

Taking Control of Your Career

I graduated with an MSN and was hired into a new grad residency program to work on a neurosurgical unit. After two years of working in neuro, my interests started to change and I desired an opportunity to explore other areas of nursing, especially critical care.

I saw an ICU opening where four training positions were available for in-house staff, and I applied. I received a call from the ICU manager and was told they had a great desire to bring me aboard as a transfer. My manager, however, was not willing to give me up quite yet and made it her purpose to intervene. Not long after, I received another call stating that I was not quite ready for the position and I should try next time. I came to find out that this same thing had already occurred to multiple other RN colleagues, some with four or five years experience on our floor.

I thought to myself: I can either stick around and try again next time, and thus allow my future career to be determined by someone else (the manager), or I can find another job elsewhere and move on to experience new areas of nursing.

Not long after this incident, I left this hospital and have never looked back. I don't regret my decision in the least. I was given a great opportunity to learn and develop as an RN in a wonderful environment, and I am utterly thankful for such a chance. I am also thankful to my new manager who has supported me in many ways.

My suggestion? Even in a poor economy where new grads are struggling to get into acute care settings, once you gain a few years of experience, seek out what you want. Don't let others determine your career path for you. Those same people have developed their own paths. Every person has this right. Always do your best, look forward and follow your bliss. Who knows, maybe you'll also find a new environment or specialty where you will thrive.

Nursing is full of opportunities! Just work hard and keep seeking. The different areas you work in can only make you a better nurse over the years. Think of it as a role-play game where you are building a character and must develop certain traits, skills and knowledge over time.

Nursing is no different.

Jeremy Weed, MSN, RN
Graduated 2008

Nursing is a career with many possibilities. If your current situation isn't rewarding – leave the job, not the profession.

Designing Your Road Map for Success

As a new graduate, I was accepted into an eight-week new grad ICU internship. This program consisted of six weeks of didactic education, combined with a one-to-one preceptorship in the ICU. The internship prepared me very well for my role as an ICU staff nurse. The following year, I was asked to be a preceptor for a new grad in the upcoming internship program.

I loved teaching/precepting and was thrilled when asked to teach a section of the ICU internship curriculum. My topic was hemodynamic monitoring interpretation and included assisting with insertion of lines and managing patients with these lines.

This experience confirmed my love of teaching, and I soon enrolled in a graduate program to earn my MSN with a focus in nursing education. Each semester, 135 clinical hours were required. One semester, I completed my clinical hours in the education department of a local community hospital. This department provided education for new hire nurses as well as on-going requirements for staff, such as CPR renewal and other competencies. I loved this experience and set the career goal of obtaining a position in a hospital education department as an educator. However, these positions were often difficult to come by and usually filled by RNs with many years of nursing experience.

One day during a break at work, I was skimming through the course offerings from my hospital's education department. There was an upcoming class offered through the National Nursing Staff Development Organization designed to prepare participants for the staff development educator certification exam. The goals and objectives of the class were exactly what I wanted to pursue.

Even though the course was designed for experienced educators, I didn't let that stop me. I immediately signed up for the course, knowing it was way too premature for me to take the exam, but I wanted exposure to the content of the new career path I was pursuing.

The course was three days long. On my first day, I quickly realized that almost the entire audience consisted of experienced nurse educators who were taking the course either to prep for the exam or to increase their knowledge in their specialty area.

Over the three-day course, I got to know these educators quite well through small group assignments and during breaks and lunch periods. I learned about their roles in the hospital and in turn, they learned about me – that I was currently working in the ICU, was pursuing my master's degree in nursing with education as a focus, and most importantly, that I was interested in a career as a hospital educator.

About a week after the course, one of the educators called to inform me that a position was opening up for a part-time educator at our sister hospital. I immediately applied for the job. Due to my past experiences of teaching/precepting in the new grad ICU internship, and because I was enrolled in the master's program, I was hired for the job. The selection process was very competitive, but I'm sure that knowing several people on the interview panel, who attended the three-day training course with me, was definitely a plus.

I loved my job as a hospital educator. I ended up working with and becoming very good friends with the educators I met during the three-day prep course. I highly recommend that once you discover your interests in the many fields you can pursue as an RN, expose yourself to the role as much as possible and network with colleagues in this specialty area. In the end, it will open doors for many opportunities to come.

Veanne O'Neill, MSN, RN
Graduated 1986

Find your path; create and seize opportunities!

Dreams

This is the story of a young woman who wanted to become a nurse. She wanted to be an RN more than anything in the world. She wanted to enter nursing school after she graduated from high school, but her dream was interrupted by a bittersweet tragedy – the loss of her mother in childbirth and the arrival of a baby sister.

Her dream was set aside as she stayed home to care for her family and little sister. Several years later, she married and had children of her own. Raising her family took time and energy that did not include following her dream.

When she was in her forties, she had an opportunity to become an LVN. A step in the right direction! She was back on track to realizing her dream of becoming an RN. A decade later, she received a scholarship to an RN program. Her excitement was beyond measure. Then it was dashed when she was challenged by others: "How could you take the place of a younger student, someone who had more years to give back to the nursing profession?"

She held onto her dream, in spite of the criticism and challenges. She became an RN. Her dream!

After graduation, she worked at a state mental hospital on the male medical ward. This was a tough job – definitely not for the faint of heart. She became the head nurse and worked diligently to set standards of care for their unit. She focused on teamwork with her employees. They loved her enthusiasm. She loved nursing.

She went on for another decade, working at a Catholic girls' college and at a health center, responding to emergencies of the residents. At 75 she hung up her cap! It was time to stop working.

Who is this person?

She was my mother, affectionately known as *Amazing Grace* by her family, friends and co-workers. She was a great nurse. She had the gift of making everyone she came in contact with feel special – this was one of her most cherished attributes.

Why tell the story of *Amazing Grace?* Because this story is also about each of us and our dreams for our profession. It's about our struggles and challenges.

If she were here today, I know my mother would wish us the following:

The courage to hold onto our dreams and never lose sight of our goals.

The tenacity to not be discouraged by criticism and challenges. When we know in our hearts that we are on the correct path – hold our heads high, shoulders back and march forward.

When we've been given a gift – whether it's a scholarship, promotion, degree or new position – may we remember to give back with our time and talents as our careers progress.

May we all keep the passion for nursing in our hearts through the good times and the challenging times.

May we never lose sight of our dreams!

Beth Gardner, MS, RN
2011 ACNL President
Graduated 1962

YOU have the power to make your dreams come true!

Afterword

Putting It All Together: Thriving as an RN!

"Nursing's role is to save the future of health care!"
Florence Wald, MN, MS, RN, FAAN

Throughout this book, we've provided information, resources and tools to help you successfully transition to your new role as an RN and thrive in your first nursing job!

Your adventure as a nurse is just beginning. As the inspiring stories from our contributors have shown, it promises to be an amazing journey, with many triumphant and rewarding experiences. But at times, the road may be rough and rocky. If that happens – don't give up! Remind yourself of the reasons you chose nursing as a career. Think about the lives you've touched and what important work you're doing as an RN. Use your resources, including the knowledge and skills you've gained from this book, to help you work through the difficult times.

Here are some important points to remember:

• As an RN, you are a professional! Understand what it means to be a professional and practice to that standard.

• Learning is a lifelong process. You don't need to know everything on your first day.

• Ask questions if you don't know something. Asking questions and verifying information will build your knowledge and reduce errors.

• Effective communication is one of the essential skills to help you be successful, both professionally and personally. Strive to improve your abilities as a communicator.

• A key component of effective communication and delegation is listening.

• As an RN, you have a powerful voice. Use it to advocate for your patients and speak up when something is wrong.

• Trust your instincts and intuition. If something doesn't feel right, stop and question it.

278 Surviving and Thriving

- One of your most important early relationships is with your preceptor. Set goals with your preceptor and communicate frequently about your needs and progress. If your relationship with your preceptor isn't working and can't be fixed – talk to your manager. A change in preceptors may be needed.

- Errors are a significant threat to the safety of our patients. If you make an error, report it. If you discover an error, talk about it. Develop strategies you can use to reduce your chances of making errors.

- Look for ways to improve patient care. If the evidence supports a better and/or safer practice, utilize it and bring it to the attention of your colleagues.

- Maintain patient confidentiality at all times.

- Know the symptoms of compassion fatigue. Strive to attain work/life balance.

- As you progress in your career, look for mentors to help you on your journey.

- Join a professional organization and get involved.

- If a job isn't right for you – leave the job, not the profession.

And always believe in yourself and the profession of nursing!

Nursing has been an incredibly rewarding career for us! Throughout this book, we've shared many stories from our nursing journeys. Now we'd like to end *Surviving and Thriving* by sharing two more stories with you – our best days in nursing.

Pat's Best Day in Nursing:

Jimmy's Long Journey to Healing

My best day in nursing started about six months before the actual day arrived. I was working in a 10-bed adult/pediatric ICU as a relief charge nurse on the p.m. shift. One evening, we received a call from the emergency department telling us that a young gunshot victim was on his way to surgery and would be admitted to our unit post-operatively.

Knowing the gunshot wound was to the patient's face, we prepared for the worst. About an hour before our shift ended, Jimmy, a beautiful 9 year-old boy, was wheeled into the unit accompanied by the anesthesiologist, neurosurgeon and his parents. There wasn't a single mark on Jimmy's face because the bullet went through his right nare. But the evidence of his injury was apparent by the large turban around his head from the craniotomy that was just performed in the OR.

We quickly went to work assessing Jimmy, reviewing physician orders and checking his IVs and ventilator settings. Soon after Jimmy's parents left, the surgeon returned to reinforce that he didn't expect his young patient to make it through the night. Although the bullet was a small caliber, it had done considerable damage to Jimmy's brain. We were to keep him comfortable and allow his family to say goodbye.

To our surprise when we arrived the next day, Jimmy was still our patient. Days turned into weeks as we slowly began to see subtle changes in Jimmy. The entire team was ecstatic. His family never wavered in their belief that Jimmy would wake up. Their compassion, love and unshakable faith were contagious. Soon we all caught the "Jimmy can recover" bug. About four weeks later, Jimmy opened his eyes. Then a few days later, he smiled – that was all we needed!

Working closely with his family, we began to outline Jimmy's road to recovery. We attempted to create a healing environment where his parents could visit, interact and work with us to bring Jimmy back. We learned that Jimmy loved a television program featuring a very attractive actress. We hung pictures of her on the ceiling and at the foot of his bed. We began dressing Jimmy in t-shirts picturing this actress. The unit had only one TV, so every Wednesday evening we would drag it to Jimmy's bedside so he could watch her TV show.

Finally, Jimmy was breathing on his own and following simple commands. It was time for him to be transferred to pediatrics. We held several team meetings to be sure the handoff to the peds unit would be smooth. While on peds, Jimmy continued to make progress and was eventually transferred to a pediatric rehab unit.

One afternoon in late spring, I was standing in the hallway outside the ICU talking to the environmental staff about a safety issue. I noticed a short-statured woman walking hand-in-hand with a young boy, heading in the direction of the cords that were draped across the hall. I was about to tell them to wait until I cleared a path, when the boy started running. He jumped over the cords and straight into my arms, almost knocking me over. It was Jimmy, our beautiful young patient who six months earlier wasn't expected to live.

On that day, I knew we had made a difference! We did what we do best – providing excellent nursing care in a therapeutic, healing environment while working as equal members of the interdisciplinary team. To this day, I carry a piece of Jimmy in my heart!

Brenda's Best Day in Nursing:

Beating the Odds!

I've had many wonderful memories from my 22 years as an RN, but my best day in nursing happened just as this book was about to go to print. On my best day as an RN, I wasn't working as a nurse – I didn't have my stethoscope, syringes, bandage scissors, penlight – or any other tools of the trade I would carry with me when providing patient care. My best day as a nurse occurred when I entered a patient's room on the cardiac floor where I had previously worked for many years. My dear friend, Connie, got out of her bed, took a few steps, called me by name and hugged me.

You're probably thinking: *That's your best day in nursing?* Yes, it certainly was!

Just 16 days previously, Connie was in the ICU, intubated and unresponsive after suffering cardiac arrest due to an episode of ventricular fibrillation while at home. Her husband didn't know CPR, but the EMS dispatcher gave him basic instructions over the telephone. When the paramedics arrived, they were able to shock her into a sinus rhythm, although she remained unresponsive. When she got to the ED, she went into V-tach and was once again defibrillated. Therapeutic hypothermia was quickly initiated so that Connie's brain would require less oxygen, hopefully minimizing the damage to her brain cells.

On day 4, both the neurologist and intensivist warned that it was highly unlikely Connie would recover beyond her vegetative state. In spite of this, the physicians and nurses continued to provide the best care possible. Her family and friends stayed by her bedside. In the early morning of day 7, she woke up and pulled out her endotracheal tube. Day by day, Connie could talk a little more, gained more control over her movements and began to recognize people. On day 13, she picked up the phone at 3 a.m., dialed her home number and told her husband she was "bored."

Tests showed no damage to her heart or brain. *Why did she go into V-fib?* It could have been her low potassium level of 2.4 when she was admitted to the hospital. Or perhaps it was an irritable ectopic focus in her ventricle that went awry. The physicians say we'll never know for sure.

On day 15, Connie was transferred to my old cardiac unit after placement of an implantable cardioverter-defibrillator (ICD). Now it's day 16, and her husband and I are sitting at her bedside while my former colleagues provide nursing care and patient education in preparation for her discharge the following day.

I can't help but reflect on how many professionals played a role in

Connie's recovery – the EMS dispatcher and paramedics; every physician and nurse who delivered the best care possible; and the other interdisciplinary team members, including occupational therapy, physical therapy, social services and chaplaincy. And let's not forget all the love, prayers and positive thoughts from the people who love her and rushed to her bedside.

But most importantly, this incident is a reminder to me of the amazing power of the human body and spirit to heal itself – if we provide the optimal circumstances for this healing to take place.

Yes indeed, this was my best day as a nurse!

We wish you much success and happiness in nursing! YOU are the future of our profession. We welcome you with open arms and wish you a long and prosperous career. Never forget what an honor and privilege it is to be an RN!

Brenda Brozek, MAOL, RN

Patricia McFarland, MS, RN, FAAN

Glossary

Accountable Care Organization (ACO) A health care organization characterized by a payment and care delivery model. This organization seeks to tie provider reimbursements to quality metrics and reductions in the total cost of care for an assigned population of patients.

Benchmarking A method of comparing performance using identified quality indicators across institutions or disciplines.

Bullying Someone who knowingly, deliberately and persistently abuses the rights of others to gain control of a situation and the individual(s) involved.

Clinical Judgment An application of clinical reasoning whereby the nurse knows why an intervention is needed, is able to perform the intervention competently, and can justify the clinical decision; allowing the clinician to fit his or her knowledge and experience to an individual patient (individual needs, history, etc.).

Clinical Reasoning An in-depth mental process of analysis and evaluation of knowledge and skills; the process of arriving at the problem identification (diagnosis).

Competence A registered nurse is considered competent when they consistently demonstrate the ability to transfer scientific knowledge from social, biological and physical sciences in applying the nursing process.

Critical Pathways Tools or guidelines that direct care by identifying expected outcomes.

Critical Thinking Actively conceptualizing, analyzing, applying, synthesizing and evaluating information.

Dashboards A combination of graphics and numbers to quickly display important data elements.

Deep Dive A tool to advance change and innovation in which a particular area is selected for observation in multiple ways. Workflows, photos, interviews and observations are gathered by a team to analyze.

Disruptive Behavior (also called incivility, or lateral or horizontal violence) Intimidating and disruptive behaviors consist of overt actions, such as verbal outbursts and physical threats, and covert activities that include uncooperative attitude, gossiping, withholding information and ostracism. Behaviors can extend outside the workplace and can occur in person or in cyberspace.

Evidence-Based Practice (EBP) The integration of best clinical practice, research evidence, nursing expertise, and the values and preferences of the individuals, families and communities who are served.

Failure to Rescue The avoidable death of a patient.

Gross Negligence Considered the extreme departure from the standard of care, which under similar circumstances, would have ordinarily been exercised by a competent RN.

Handoffs Accurate information about a patient's general care plan, treatment, service, current conditions and any recent or anticipated changes provided by one health care provider to another when the patient changes physical location (such as from one unit to another) or changes health care providers.

Iatrogenic Error Adverse effects or complications resulting from medical treatment or advice.

Joint Commission (JC) A private, nonprofit organization that evaluates and accredits hospitals and other health care organizations. The range of organizations extend from acute care hospitals to providing home care, behavioral health care, ambulatory care and long-term care services.

Just Culture A learning environment where errors are investigated and systems corrected to reduce future mistakes by examining choices the individual made in relation to the error.

Lean A quality improvement methodology focusing on eliminating waste while focusing on what customers consider quality.

Lean Six Sigma Quality improvement methodology resulting from the combination of the individual Lean and Six Sigma programs.

Magnet Recognition Program Recognition by the American Nurses Credentialing Center that a health care organization provides quality nursing care based on Magnet standards.

Never Events A list compiled by the National Quality Forum, of preventable adverse health events that should *never* occur in the heatlh care setting. Examples of *Never Events* include: surgery on the wrong body part; death or serious disability associated with a fall occurring in a health care institution; and a stage 3 or 4 pressure ulcer acquired after admission to a health care facility.

Onboarding The early processes of socializing nurses into the workplace to achieve optimal employee engagement.

Plan-Do-Study-Act (PDSA) A continuous quality improvement model consisting of a logical sequence of four repeated steps: Plan, Do, Study (Check) and Act.

Rapid Response Team (RRT) A team of health care clinicians (physicians, nurses, respiratory therapists and others) and experts in critical care, who come to the bedside to assist staff in making rapid decisions when a patient's condition is deteriorating.

Risk Management A program that seeks to identify and eliminate potential safety hazards, thereby reducing patient injuries.

Sentinel Event An unanticipated event in a health care setting that results in death or serious physical or psychological injury to a person, not related to the natural course of the patient's illness.

Six Sigma A set of strategies, techniques and tools for process improvement. Six Sigma seeks to improve the quality of process outputs by identifying and removing errors and minimizing variability.

TeamSTEPPS Team Strategies and Tools to Enhance Performance and Patient Safety is an evidence-based comprehensive system to train health care workers in the skills needed to function as a safe, effective team.

Acronyms

ACA	Affordable Care Act
ACO	Accountable Care Organization
ACNL	Association of California Nurse Leaders
AHRQ	Agency for Health Care Research and Quality
ANA	American Nurses Association
APRN	Advanced Practice Registered Nurse
BC	Board Certified
CALNOC	Collaborative Alliance for Nursing Outcomes
CMS	Center for Medicare and Medicaid Services
CPOE	Computerized Physician Order Entry
CQI	Continuous Quality Improvement
EBM	Evidence-Based Management
EBP	Evidence-Based Practice
EHR	Electronic Health Records
EMR	Electronic Medical Records
FAAN	Fellow of the American Academy of Nursing
FNI	Future of Nursing Initiative
FTR	Failure to Rescue
HAC	Hospital Acquired Condition
HCR	Health Care Reform
HHS	US Department of Health and Human Services
HIPAA	Health Insurance Portability and Accountability Act
IHI	Institute for Healthcare Improvement
IOM	Institute of Medicine
IPPS	Inpatient Prospective Payment System
IRB	Institutional Review Board
JC / TJC	The Joint Commission
NDNQI	National Database of Nursing Quality Indicators
NIH	National Institute of Health
NQF	National Quality Forum
PHR	Personal Health Record
PI	Performance Improvement
QI	Quality Improvement
QSEN	Quality and Safety Education for Nurses
RM	Risk Management
RRT	Rapid Response Team
RWJF	Robert Wood Johnson Foundation
SBAR	Situation Background Assessment Recommendation
TCAB	Transforming Care at Bedside
TQM	Total Quality Management

References and Resources

Chapter 1 – What to Expect: Your Growth as a Professional Nurse

Benner, P. (2001). *From novice to expert: Excellence and power in clinical nursing*. Upper Saddle River, New Jersey: Prentice Hall Health.

Cardin, S., and Rodgers, C. (1989). *Personnel management in critical care nursing*. Baltimore, Maryland: Williams & Wilkin, 59-70.

Duchscher, J. B. (2008). A process of becoming: The stages of new nursing graduate professional role transition. *The Journal of Continuing Education in Nursing*, Vol.39, No. 10, 441-450.

Nicoteri, J. A. (1998). Critical thinking skills. *American Journal of Nursing*, Vol. 98, No.10, 62, 64-65.

Pellico, L. H., Brewer, C. S., and Kovner, C. T. (2009). What newly licensed registered nurses have to say about their first experiences. *Nursing Outlook*, Vol. 57, No. 4, 194-203.

Smith, M. E. (2007). From student to practicing nurse: How institutions, managers, and colleagues can ease the transitions. *American Journal of Nursing*, Vol. 107, No. 7, 72A-72D.

Chapter 2 – Paving the Road: Preceptors, Mentors and Role Models

Grossman, S. (2012). *Mentoring in nursing: A dynamic and collaborative process*, (2nd ed.). New York, New York: Springer Publication Company, LLC.

Joel, L. A. (1997). Charged to mentor. *American Journal of Nursing*, Vol. 97, No. 2, 7.

May, L. (1980). Clinical preceptors for new nurses. *American Journal of Nursing*, Vol. 80, No. 10, 1824-1826.

Woodfine, P. (2011). Professional growth: Taking a novice nurse under your wing. *Nursing 2011*, Vol. 41, No. 9, 53-55.

Chapter 3 – Defining Your Role as an RN: Important Resources to Guide Your Practice

American Association of College of Nursing (2013). Hallmark of professional practice environment. Retrieved from *http://www.aacn.nche.edu/publications/white-papers/hallmarks-practice-environment*

American Nurses Association (2003). *Nursing's social policy statement*, (3rd ed.). Silver Springs, Maryland.

American Nurses Association (2008). *Code of ethics for nurses with interpretive statements*, (Reissued 2010). Silver Springs, Maryland.

American Nurses Association (2010). *Scope and standards of practice*, (2nd ed.). Silver Springs, Maryland.

Barter, M., and McFarland, P., (2001). BSN by 2010: A California Initiative. *The Journal of Nursing Administration*, Vol. 3, No. 31, 141-144.

Black, B. and Chitty, K. (2007). *Professional nursing concepts & challenges*, Fifth Edition. St. Louise, Missouri: Saunders Elsevier.

Clavelle, J., and Drenkard, K. (2012). Transformational leadership practices of chief nursing officers in magnet organizations. *The Journal of Nursing Administration*, Vol.42, No. 4, 195-201.

D'Amour, D., Dubois, C., Dery, J., Clarke, S., Tchouaket, E., Blais, R., and Rivard, M. (2012). Measuring actual scope of nursing practice. *The Journal of Nursing Administration*, Vol.42, No. 5, 248-255.

Institute of Medicine (2011). *The future of nursing: Leading change, advancing health*. Washington DC: Institute of Medicine and National Academies Press.

National Council of State Boards of Nursing (n.d.). Nurse Licensure Compact Fact sheet: What nurse employers need to know. Retrieved from: http://www.ncsbn.org/2010_NLCA_factsheet_Employers_FI-NAL_2.pdf

Nightingale, F. (1860). *Notes on nursing*, (Reprinted first American ed.) New York, New York: D. Appleton Company.

O'Rourke, M. (2009). RN's professional role is established by law. *BRN Report*, Fall/Winter. Retrieved from: http://www.rn.ca.gov/pdfs/regulations/npr-i-00.pdf

O'Rourke, M. and White, A. (2011). Professional role clarity and competency in health care staffing: The missing pieces. *Nursing Economics$*, Vol. 29, No. 4, 183-188.

Poe, L. (2008). Nursing regulation, the nurse licensure compact, and nurse administrators – working together for patient safety. *Nursing Administration Quarterly*, Vol. 32, No. 4, 267-272.

Porter-O'Grady, T., and Malloch, K. (2006). *Introduction to evidence-based practice in nursing and health care*. Burlington, Massachusetts: Jones & Bartlett Learning.

Russell, K. (2012). Nurse practice acts guide and govern nursing practice. *Journal of Nursing Regulation*, Vol.3, No. 3, 36-42.

Shaffer, L., Johnson K., and Guinn, C. (2010). Remedying role confusion: Differentiating RN and LPN roles. *American Nurse Today*, Vol. 5, No.3, 61-63.

Sullivan, E. (2012). *Effective leadership and management in nursing*, (8th ed.). Boston, Massachusetts: Pearson.

Ulrich, C. (2012). *Nursing ethics in everyday practice.* Indianapolis, Indiana: Sigma Theta Tau International – Honor Society of Nursing.

BellaOnLine – *The Voice of Woman – Career Training Site.* Retrieved from: http://www.bellaonline.com/articles/art48951.asp

Chapter 4 – Communication Skills: The Foundation of Your Success as an RN

Facente, A. (2010). Toward cultural competence: One hospital's effort to create a culturally sensitive health care community. *American Journal of Nursing*, Vol. 110, No. 12, 52-55.

Gerace, L., and Salimbene, S. (2010). Culturally diverse nursing staff: Working together. *Continuing Education.* Retrieved from: http://www.continuingeducation.com/course/cme402/cultural-competence-for-to-days-nurses-part-five-culturally-diverse-nursing-staff-working-together

Grossman, D, and Taylor, R. (1995). Cultural diversity on the unit: A little extra care in communicating with nurses of different cultural backgrounds can pay surprising dividends in quality and morale. *American Journal of Nursing*, Vol. 95, No. 2, 64-67.

Lincoln, B. (2010). *Reflections from common ground...cultural awareness in healthcare.* Eau Claire, Wisconsin: PHC Publishing Group.

Lipson, J. G., and Dibble, S. (2007). *Culture and clinical care.* UCSF Nursing Press. http://nursing.ucsf.edu/ucsf-nursing-press-culture-clinical-care

Maddron, T. (2002). *Living your colors, practical wisdom for life, love, work and play.* New York, New York: Warner Books, Inc.

Miller, S., Wackman, D., Nunnally, E., and Miller, P. (1992). *Connecting with self and others.* Littleton, CO: Interpersonal Communication Programs.

Miscisin, M. (2001). *Showing our true colors.* Riverside, California: True Colors Inc. Publishing.

Miscisin, M. (n.d.). The gift of feedback. Retrieved from: http://www.positivelymary.com/Free-Stuff/Feedback-Article.htm

Pagana, K. (2012). How to keep your communication professional. *American Nurse Today*, Vol. 7, No. 9, 56-58.

Zemke, R., Rainses, C., and Filipczak, B. (2000). *Generations at work.* New York, New York: AMA Publications.

Chapter 5 – Effective Communication: Strategies for Challenging Situations

American Nurses Association (2012). *Bullying in the workplace: Reversing a culture,* (2012 ed.). Silver Springs, Maryland:

Cuddy A. (2012). Your body language shapes who you are. Retrieved from http://www.ted.comtalks/any_cuddy_your_body_language_shapes_who_you_are.html

Diamond, S. (2010). *Getting more, how to negotiate to achieve your goals in the real world.* New York, New York: Crown Publishing Group.

Horn, S. (2002). *Take the bully by the horns.* New York, New York: St. Martin's Press.

Patterson, K. Grenny, J., McMillan, R., and Switzler, A. (2002). *Crucial conversations, tools for talking when stakes are high.* New York, New York: McGraw-Hill.

Dizik, A. (2012). Six ways to deal with criticism at work. Retrieved from http://online.wsj.com/article/SB10001424052702303753904577452330484680636.html?KEYWORDS=Six+ways+to+deal+with+Criticism+at+work

Gesssler, R., Rosenstein, A., and Ferron, L. (2012). *How to handle disruptive physician behaviors: Find out the best way to respond if you're the target.* American Nurse Today, Vol. 7, No. 11, 8-10.

Hughes, D. J, (2011). The 3 R's for dealing with workplace bullying. Retrieved from http://endonurse.com/PrinterFriendly.aspx?id

Maxfield, D., Grenny, J., Lavandero, R., and Groah, L. (n.d.). The silent treatment: Why safety tools and checklists aren't enough to save lives. Retrieved from http://www.aacn.org/WD/hwe/docs/the-silent-treatment.pdf

Maxfield, D., Grenny, J., McMillian, R., Patterson, K., and Switzler, A. (2005). Silence Kills: The seven crucial conversation for healthcare. Retrieved from http://www.aacn.org/WD/practice/docs/publicpolicy/silencekills.pdf

Nurse.com (2013). Study measures impact in verbal abuse on new RN's. Retrieved from http://news.nurse.com/article/20130618/ML02/306180047

Rosenstein, A. H., and O'Daniel, M. (2008). A survey of the impact of disruptive behavior and communication defects on patient safety. *The Joint Commission Journal on Quality and Patient Safety*. Vol. 34, No. 8, 464-471.

The Joint Commission (2008). Behaviors that undermine a culture of safety. Retrieved from http://www.jointcommission.org/sentinel_event_ alert_issue_40_behaviors_that_undermine_a_culture_of_safety

Chapter 6 – Delegation: Empowerment and Accountability

American Nurse Association (2005). *Working with others: A position paper*. Silver Springs, Maryland: American Nurses Publishing.

American Nurse Association and the National Council of State Boards of Nursing (2013). *Joint statement of delegation*. Silver Springs, Maryland: American Nurses Publishing.

Davidson, S. B., Scott, R., and Minarik, P. (1999). Thinking critically about delegation. *American Journal of Nursing*, Vol.99, No. 6, 61-62.

Parkman, C., A. (1996). Delegation: Are you doing it right? *American Journal of Nursing*, Vol.96, No. 9, 43-48.

Porter-O'Grady, T. and Malloch, K. (2013). *Leadership in nursing practice*. Burlington, Massachusetts: Jones & Bartlett Learning.

Whitman, M. (2004). Return and report: Establishing accountability in delegation. *American Journal of Nursing*, Vol.104, No. 11, 76.

Chapter 7 – Opportunity or Uncertainty: Successfully Managing Change

Bridges, W. (2004). *Transition, making sense of life's changes*. Cambridge, Massachusetts: Perseus Books.

Kotter, J. (1996). *Leading change*. Cambridge, Massachusetts: Harvard Business School Press.

Kubler-Ross, E. (1969). *On death and dying*. New York, New York: Macmillan Publishing Company.

Lewin, K. (1951). *Field theory in social science*. New York, New York: Harper & Row.

McGovern, W., and Rodgers, J. (1986). Change theory. *American Journal of Nursing*, Vol. 86, No. 5, 566-567.

Chapter 8 – Quality and Patient Safety: You Can Make a Difference!

Albanese, M., Evans, D., Schantz, C., Bowen, M., Moffa, J., Piesieski, P., and Polomano, R. (2010). Engaging clinical nurses in quality and performance improvement activities. *Nursing Administration Quarterly,* Vol. 34, No. 3, 226-245.

Amer, K. (2013). *Quality and safety for transformational nursing – Core competencies.* Boston, Massachusetts: Pearson.

American Association of Colleges of Nursing (n.d.). *Hallmarks of quality and patient safety – Recommended baccalaureate competencies and curricular guidelines to assure high quality and safe patient care.* Washington, D.C.

American Nurses Association (1995). *Nursing care report card for acute care.* Washington. D.C.

Castner, J., Foltz-Ramos, K., Schwarts, D., and Ceravolo, D. (2012). A leadership challenge – staff nurse perceptions after an organizational Team STEPPS initiative. *The Journal of Nursing Administration,* Vol. 42, No. 10, 467-472.

Colevas, A., and Rempe, B. (2011). Nurse-sensitive indicators: Integral to the Magnet Journey. *American Nurse Today,* Vol. 6, No. 1, 39-41.

Cook, A. F., and Hoas, H., Guttmannova, K., and Joyner J. C. (2004). An error by any other name. *American Journal of Nursing,* Vol. 104, No. 6, 32-43.

Davis, P., Hensley, S. L., Muzik, L., Comeau, O., Bell, L., Carroll, A R., Sathre, R. . . . Brumfield, V. (2012). Enhancing RN professional engagement and contribution: An innovative competency and clinical advancement program. *Nurse Leader,* Vol. 10, No. 3, 34-39.

Fagan, M. (2012). Techniques to improve patient safety in hospitals. *The Journal of Nursing Administration,* Vol. 42, No. 9, 426-430.

Finkelman, A., and Kenner, C. (2012). Teaching IMO – *Implication of the Institute of Medicine reports for nursing education* (3ed.). Silver Springs, Maryland.

Gorzeman, J. (2008). Balancing just culture with regulatory standards. *Nursing Administration Quarterly,* Vol. 32, No. 4, 308-311.

Greising, C. and Foster, S. (2012). Transforming a culture for safety and quality. *Hospitals & Health Networks,* Vol. 86, No. 09, 14.

Hughes, C., Chang, Y., and Mark, B. (2009). Quality and strength of patient safety climate on medical-surgical units. *The Journal of Nursing Administration,* Vol. 42, No. 10, 27-36.

Institute of Medicine (1999). *To err is human: Building a safer health system.* Washington DC: Institute of Medicine and National Academies Press.

Institute of Medicine (2001). *Crossing the quality chasm: A new health system for the 21st century.* Washington D.C: Institute of Medicine and National Academies Press.

Institute of Medicine (2003). *Health professions education: A bridge to quality.* Washington D.C: Institute of Medicine and National Academies Press.

Institute of Medicine (2011). *The future of nursing. Leading change, advancing health.* Washington DC: Institute of Medicine and National Academies Press.

Leach, L. S., Mayo, A., and O'Rourke, M. (2010). How RNs rescue patients: a qualitative study of RNs' perceived involvement in rapid response teams. *Quality & Safety in Health Care,* 19: 1-4, dol: 10.1136/qshc.2008.030494

Studer Group, (2013). *Valued-based purchasing at a glance – Fiscal year 2013 and your organization.* Retrieved from https://az414866.vo.msecnd.net/cmsroot/studergroup/media/studergroup/pages/our-impact/hcahps/vbp/2013_vbp_at_a_glance.pdf

The Joint Commission (2013). *Facts about the national patient safety goals.* Retrieved from http://www.jointcommission.org/standards_information/npsgs.aspx

Chapter 9 – Endless Possibilities: Looking Beyond Your 1st Job

Boyle, D. A. (2011). Countering compassion fatigue: A requisite agenda. *The Online Journal of Issues in Nursing,* Vol. 16, No. 1, Manuscript 2. Retrieved from http://www.nursingworld.org/MainMenuCategories/ANAMarketplace/ANAPeriodicals/OJIN/TableofContents/Vol-16-2011/No1-Jan-2011/Countering-Compassion-Fatigue.html

Lombardo, B., and Eyre, C. (2011). Compassion fatigue: A nurse's primer. *The Online Journal of Issues in Nursing,* Vol. 16, No. 1, Manuscript 3. Retrieved from http://www.nursingworld.org/MainMenuCategories/ANAMarketplace/ANAPeriodicals/OJIN/TableofContents/Vol-16-2011/No1-Jan-2011/Compassion-Fatigue-A-Nurses-Primer.html

Murphy, K. (2010). Combating compassion fatigue. *Nursing Made Incredibly Easy,* Vol. 8, No. 4, 4. Retrieved from http://journals.lww.com/nursingmadeincrediblyeasy/Fulltext/2010/07000/Combating_compassion_fatigue.1.aspx

Sandberg, S. (2013). *Lean in.* New York, New York: Alfred A. Knopf.

Websites

For additional information we found these websites to be most helpful and informative:

Agency for Healthcare Research and Quality (AHRQ) *www.ahrq.gov*

American Nurses Association (ANA) *www.nursingworld.org*

American Nurses Credentialing Center (ANCC) *www.nursingcredentialing.org*

Association of California Nurse Leaders (ACNL) *www.acnl.org*

Centers for Medicare & Medicaid (CMS) *www.cms.gov*

Cochrane Collaborative Library *www.cochrane.org*

Collaborative Alliance for Nursing Outcomes (CALNOC) *www.calnoc.org*

Institute for Healthcare Improvement (IHI) *www.ihi.org*

Institute of Medicine (IOM) *www.iom.edu*

Joanna Briggs Institute *www.joannabriggs.edu.au*

The Joint Commission (JC) *www.jointcommision.org*

National Council of State Board Nursing (NCSBN) *www.ncsbn.org*

National Database of Nursing Quality Indicators (NDNQI) *www.nursingquality.org.*

National Quality Forum (NQF) *www.qualityforum.org*

Sigma Theta Tau International *www.nursingsociety.org*

My Notes...

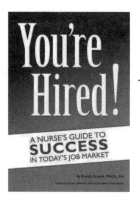